Keep Moving!

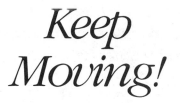

Keep Moving!

It's Aerobic Dance

Esther Kan
SOLANO COLLEGE

Minda Goodman Kraines
MISSION COLLEGE

Mayfield Publishing Company

Dedicated to our husbands,
Michael Kan and Guy Kraines.
Without their patience, support, and love,
this book could not have been completed.

---

10   9   8   7   6   5   4

Credits: Kelly Ann Garcia, Michael R. Kan, and Julia Kimsey
appear on the cover with Esther Kan and, along with
Karen Stenger, modelled for the photographs used to create the
sketches in this book. These photographs were generously
provided by Mike Jory.

Photographs on pages 12 and 18
were provided by Peter Anning.

Mayfield Publishing Company
1240 Villa Street
Mountainview, California 94041

Sponsoring editor: James Bull
Manuscript editor: Eva Marie Strock
Managing editor: Pat Herbst
Art director: Cynthia Bassett
Designer: Albert Burkhardt
Illustrator: Mary Burkhardt
Cover photograph: Tim Davis Photography
Production manager: Cathy Willkie
Compositor: G & S Typesetters, Inc.
Printer and binder: Malloy Lithographing

Contents

CHAPTER 8

Body Toning 63

CHAPTER 9

Cool-down 79

CHAPTER 10

Stress and Relaxation 91

CHAPTER 11

Body Composition 95

Foreword

Keep Moving! It's Aerobic Dance is an excellent book for anyone interested in fitness. I've been teaching Aerobic Dance since 1976. It has been my pleasure and reward to watch it grow into a multi-million-dollar-a-year industry . . . You can't stop a good program! There were 28 million people participating in Aerobic Dance classes in 1985, and the number keeps growing.

Naturally, in any field that is growing at such a tremendous rate, it is difficult to keep participants well informed. That is what this book aims to do—provide good information.

Esther Kan and Minda Goodman Kraines have produced a well-written, practical, and educational book—truly one of the best I've read on the subject. They completely break down all the elements of aerobic dance, from why an aerobic workout is important, to what the various components of an aerobic dance class are. Nutrition, body composition, injury prevention, components of fitness, and much more are addressed in *Keep Moving! It's Aerobic Dance.*

Joanie Greggains
"Morning Stretch"

Foreword

Your personal lifestyle choices, experts say, greatly affect your health. For a long and healthy life, you need to maintain an ideal body weight, avoid smoking and substance abuse, watch your intake of saturated fats and salt, and include substantial amounts of fruits, vegetables, and fiber in your diet. Above all, you need exercise. With its intrinsic benefits and its ability to moderate many risk factors, exercise is the key to your personal health program.

At first inspection, these new prescriptions for a healthy life may seem terribly limiting and disagreeable. But no perception could be further from the truth. Health requires autonomy, personal independence, voluntary selection of options, and assumption of the power to change your own future. Good health allows you to freely experience joy, beauty, and triumph.

In this book, written with both joyous expression and scientific accuracy, Esther Kan and Minda Goodman Kraines provide the feeling as well as the substance of an important form of exercise that can help you achieve good health. Aerobic dance can help you control many specific risks to good health and at the same time provide enjoyment in its purest sense. *Keep Moving!* provides a solid, scientific background necessary for the beginning student of aerobic dance to understand what happens to the body during the early months of aerobic training. Description of the warm-ups and dances will help the beginner become familiar with unfamiliar exercises and routines that are the basis of a successful dance program.

I hope that many will read and use this book and embark successfully on new experiences.

James F. Fries, M.D.
author of *Take Care of Yourself: Consumers Guide to Medical Care*

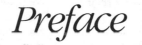

Preface

There was a time when physical exercise was a routine part of daily life. Since the invention of modern conveniences, however, we no longer physically stress our bodies in the course of our daily adventures. Therefore, we must set aside time to keep our bodies physically fit. The fitness craze, or our awareness of the need for exercise, began in the 1970s. Since then, exercise has become an accepted and integral part of daily life for many people. Aerobic exercise, in particular, has come to public attention because of evidence that it may reduce the risk of cardiovascular and respiratory disease.

Aerobic dance is one of the most popular and exhilarating forms of aerobic exercise. It combines the health and muscle toning benefits of jogging with the excitement and joy of dancing. It provides a vigorous exercise workout, while the upbeat tempo of the music creates an atmosphere of fun that is both physically and emotionally stimulating.

Aerobic dance provides all the essential advantages of a complete physical fitness program. It

- Improves the functioning of the respiratory and circulatory systems

- Strengthens the heart
- Lowers the resting heart rate
- Trims and tones the body's musculature

Aerobic dance should be pursued not only from a physical but also from an intellectual standpoint. In order to reap the full benefits of the activity, it is important for participants to know why and how aerobic dance affects the body.

Keep Moving! is a text for aerobic dance students that bridges the gap between the physical aspects and the physiological effects of a workout. It is written in a concise, lucid style, with easy-to-follow examples and illustrations. We discuss the important fitness principles and techniques that every aerobic dance student needs to know, and we present detailed descriptions of widely accepted fitness and dance exercises.

Although the focus of the text is on aerobic dance and fitness, one chapter is about posture. Chapter 5 includes a series of illustrated exercises to help students achieve correct body alignment. Instructors and students of aerobic dance will also appreciate Chapter 4, "What to Expect in an Aerobic Dance Class." There we explain what to wear and what to bring to class, the importance of regular attendance, and medical considerations, and we present a checklist for a successful class. Information such as this eliminates the need for lengthy explanation by the instructor and allows more class time for dancing.

Warm-up, aerobic dance steps, body toning, and cool-down are discussed in separate chapters. Each of these chapters contains exercises that are widely accepted aerobic dance movements. The muscle groups used in the exercises are clearly illustrated, and students are advised of precautions they should take when they perform each exercise. In a chapter on stress and relaxation, we describe relaxation exercise techniques. Also included in *Keep Moving!* is information about body composition, nutrition and diet, nonimpact and low-impact aerobic dance, and the prevention and treatment of aerobic dance injuries.

We believe that *Keep Moving!* is a valuable guide for instructors and students of aerobic dance. Our intent has been to increase your knowledge and appreciation of this popular, exhilarating activity.

For their suggestions and critical reading of an early draft of our manuscript, we wish to thank Elizabeth Brown, University of Maryland; Gail G. Evans, San Jose State University; Lorna L. Francis, San Diego State University; Barbara Jahn, University of California at Davis; Beverly McCraw, Duke University; and Janice Gudde Plastino, University of California at Irvine.

We would also like to thank Sylvia Kraines, Eleanore Goodman, Sidney Goodman, Mary Kugelman, and Phillip Sienna for helping us to see this book to its completion.

Keep moving!
Esther Kan
Minda Goodman Kraines

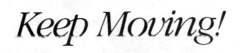

Keep Moving!

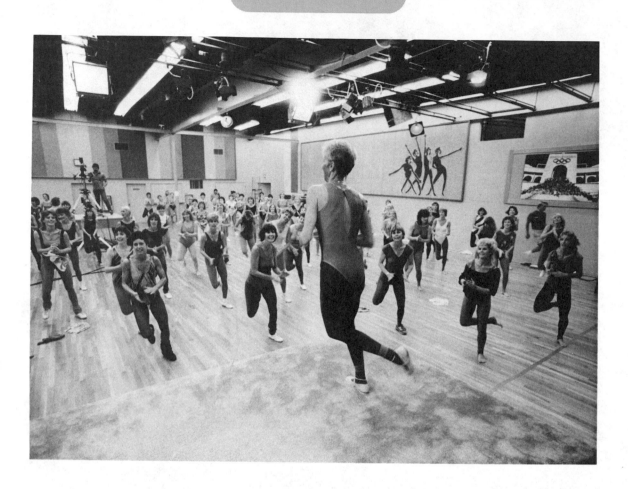

Judi Sheppard Missett, founder of Jazzercise, leading a class.

What Is Fitness?

Chapter

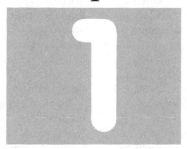

The term *fitness* is broadly used and often vaguely defined. Many people perceive health and fitness as one and the same, yet there is a definite distinction between the two concepts. Health reflects a person's state of being; it is typically viewed as the presence or absence of disease. Fitness, on the other hand, is the ability to do physical activity or to perform physical work (23).

Health and physical education experts generally agree about the expanded (but incomplete) definition of fitness as an ability to carry out daily tasks with vigor and alertness, without undue fatigue, while still maintaining ample energy to enjoy leisure-time pursuits and to meet unforeseen emergencies. However, this definition does not address the components of fitness: strength, flexibility, and endurance. It is the combination of these three components that leads to the achievement of fitness.

STRENGTH

Strength is the ability of a muscle or a group of muscles to exert a force against a resistance in one all-out effort (26). An example of such an action is the performance of one maximum lift in a weight-lifting exercise.

The body needs muscular strength for several reasons. First, strong muscles increase joint stability, which in turn makes the body joints less susceptible to injury (26). Second, improved muscle tone also helps prevent common postural problems. For example, stronger abdominal muscles can help alleviate postural problems associated with the back. Often, back problems occur because the strength in the spinal muscles is greater than that in the abdominal muscles; this muscular imbalance causes postural deviations such as lordosis, kyphosis, and even scoliosis.

Third, the body needs muscular strength because it contributes to agility, helps control the weight of the body in motion, and helps the body maneuver quickly (26). For muscular strength to be increased, the muscles must be contracted against a heavy resistance. As the muscles become stronger, the resistance applied must be increased (26) if muscular strength is to continue to increase.

FLEXIBILITY

Although flexibility is generally associated with the elasticity of muscles, the total concept of flexibility is denoted by the range of motion of a certain joint and its corresponding muscle groups. Flexibility is influenced by the structure of the joint's bones and ligaments, the amount of bulk that surrounds the joint, and the elasticity of the muscles whose tendons cross the joint (26).

The range of motion of the body's various joints is defined as *joint mobility.* Joint mobility is measured by the amount of movement that exists where two joint surfaces articulate with each other. The greater the range of motion at the joint, the more the muscles can flex and extend. This range of motion or joint mobility is specific to each joint in the body. For example, your hip joint may be extremely flexible, whereas your shoulder joint may be inflexible (35).

There are several reasons why good joint mobility and muscular elasticity should be maintained. The movement range of muscles and joints not used frequently and regularly throughout their full range of motion becomes limited. Many movement experts claim that a lack of flexibility is a cause of improper movement performance in simple motor activities such as walking and running (26). Good joint mobility and muscular elasticity can also increase resistance to muscular injury and soreness; it is the person with inflexible muscles and joints who may experience muscular soreness or who may be more easily injured during activity because of the limited range of motion (26). However, too much flexibility in certain joints, such as the weight-bearing joints of the hips, knees, or ankles, may make a person more susceptible to injury or hamper performance. Loose ligaments may allow a joint to twist abnormally, tearing the cartilage and other soft tissue. In general, it is advisable to achieve and maintain a "normal" amount of flexibility throughout the body—normal range varies with each individual.

For flexibility to be increased, the muscles must be stretched about 10 percent beyond their normal range of motion (13). As flexibility increases, the range of the stretch must also be increased.

ENDURANCE

Endurance is the ability of a muscle or group of muscles to perform work (repeated muscular contractions) for a long time. With endurance, a muscle is able to resist fatigue when a movement is repeated over and over or when a muscle is held in a static contraction (the muscle generates a motionless force for an extended time) (19).

There are two types of endurance: muscular and cardiovascular. *Muscular endurance* is the ability of local skeletal muscles to work strenuously for progressively longer periods of time without fatigue, such as during the execution of 50 sit-ups. Muscular endurance can be attained by applying overload to the muscles, either by adding weight or by increasing repetitions. But note that muscle endurance is highly specific; it will be attained only by the specific muscles exercised (26).

Cardiovascular (also called cardiorespiratory) *endurance* is the ability of the cardiovascular system (heart and blood vessels) and the respiratory system (lungs and air passages) to function efficiently during sustained, vigorous activities, such as running, swimming, and cycling. To function efficiently, the cardiorespiratory system must be able to increase both the amount of oxygen-rich blood it delivers to the working muscles and its ability to carry away carbon dioxide and other waste products. For cardiovascular endurance to be developed, a person must engage in aerobic activities that involve large muscle groups and that are continuous, rhythmic, and repetitive, such as walking, jogging, running, bicycling, skating, cross-country skiing, swimming, and aerobic dance.

AEROBIC EXERCISE VS. ANAEROBIC EXERCISE

The term *aerobic* means "with oxygen." Aerobic exercise is physical activity that utilizes oxygen for a sustained period of time (longer than 2 minutes).

During aerobic activity, the muscles being exercised use increased amounts of oxygen and produce corresponding amounts of carbon dioxide. The amount of oxygen a body can consume per minute, the *maximum oxygen uptake* or *maximum aerobic capacity,* indicates the efficiency of the heart and lungs. Maximum oxygen uptake is one of the more important factors determining human ability to sustain high-intensity exercise beyond 4 or 5 minutes (32). Thus, increased maximal oxygen uptake improves cardiovascular fitness.

When the body works at a very high intensity and cannot quickly enough deliver oxygen to the cells of the working muscles, the body's *anaerobic* ("without oxygen") processes take over and help supply the cells with energy. In anaerobic metabolism, the working muscles use the energy supplied by the combination of the breakdown of ATP (adenosine triphosphate) in the muscle cell and the secretion of the hormone epinephrine from the adrenal glands, which causes glycogen to break down to lactic acid. Exercise dependent upon anaerobic metabolism cannot be continued very long because both ATP and glycogen are in short supply in the muscle (19). Also, intense exercise cannot be continued very long due to the accumulation of lactic acid in the muscle. If there is a great accumulation of lactic acid, fatigue sets in and muscular contractions stop.

During anaerobic exercise, the body consumes excessive amounts of oxygen, leading to an oxygen deficit or debt that must be paid back (30). The oxygen debt is why labored breathing follows short and intense anaerobic activities. This oxygen debt does not occur during aerobic exercise because the cardiorespiratory system is continually supplying oxygen, which explains why aerobic exercise can be sustained for long periods of time (as in marathon running, for example), whereas anaerobic exercise (such as sprinting) is of short duration (30).

Because anaerobic exercise does not depend on an oxygen supply, it does not significantly tax the circulatory system and so is not useful in developing cardiorespiratory fitness. Aerobic exercise is the most efficient means for improving the fitness of the cardiorespiratory system because it places increased demands on the heart and lungs to deliver oxygen to the working muscles. It is the ability of the heart and lungs to deliver this oxygen that determines success in aerobic activities.

TRAINING EFFECT

The term *training effect* describes the physiological changes that occur from *regular* participation in a fitness program. To achieve a training effect and experience the benefits of exercise (whether strength, flexibility, or endurance), an individual must apply the concepts of threshold of training, overload principle, and specificity principle when exercising.

Threshold of Training

In developing physical fitness, there is a "correct" amount of exercise that will produce effective conditioning results. The *threshold of training* is the minimum amount of exercise necessary to produce improvements in physical fitness. The *fitness target zone* is within the threshold of training and the point where the benefits of exercise become counterproductive (see Chapter 3). To get optimal benefits from regular exercise, a person should exercise within the fitness target zone. Each component of fitness—strength, flexibility, and endurance—has its own threshold of training and fitness target zone. In addition, to gain fitness, a person must "overload" above the threshold of training for the exercise performed (13).

Overload Principle

For a person to experience a training effect, selected systems of the body must be subjected to loads greater than those to which they are accustomed. This is known as the *overload principle:* A body adapts to the higher performance levels and gradually increases its capacity to do more work. The principle can be summed up in this simple "rule": Do more today than you did yesterday, and do more tomorrow than you did today.

The overload principle affects the development of strength, flexibility, and endurance. For muscular strength to increase, muscles must work against a greater-than-normal load. For flexibility to increase, muscles must be stretched beyond their current length. For endurance to improve, muscles must be exposed to increasingly more sustained work. For cardiorespiratory endurance to improve, there must be an increased demand on the heart and lungs to sustain aerobic activity.

Basically, the overload principle may be applied to a fitness program in five ways:

1. Increase the number of repetitions or distance of the exercise.
2. Increase the duration or time of the exercise.
3. Increase the speed of the exercise.
4. Increase the intensity or resistance of the exercise.
5. Decrease the rest intervals between exercise.

For the cardiorespiratory system to attain a training effect, three variables of overload must be applied to the training program: intensity, duration, and frequency.

Intensity

Intensity refers to how stressful the exercise is. In the cardiorespiratory system, the intensity of the exercise should correspond to approximately 60 to 85 percent of a person's maximum heart rate (2). Exercise performed at a level below 60 percent of maximum heart rate offers few, if any, conditioning benefits. Similarly, activity at levels above 85 percent provides little added benefits and in fact may be dangerous for some people.

Duration

Duration is the length of each exercise session. For cardiorespiratory fitness to be developed, exercise should be 12 to 60 minutes of continuous activity, the time depending upon the intensity of the activity. Lower intensity activities must be performed for a longer time and are recommended for the nonathletic adult (2).

Frequency

Frequency is the number of exercise periods each week; three to five sessions a week are necessary for a training effect to be achieved (2). Even exercise of adequate intensity and duration may not effectively improve physical fitness if it is not performed regularly (2). A minimum of 8 to 12 weeks is necessary for a training effect to result.

Thus, even if the intensity, duration, and frequency are sufficient, most likely there will be no cardiorespiratory changes unless there has been participation in a continuous program for a minimum of 8 weeks.

Specificity Principle

The specificity principle (specific adaptations to imposed demands—SAID—principle) is a unifying concept that applies to all areas of fitness. It means that the human body adapts specifically to the demands placed upon it. For example, strength training induces specific strength adaptations, but strength training does *not* develop cardiorespiratory fitness. Only training involving aerobic exercises produces specific endurance training adaptations (32).

The specificity principle also applies to each body part. If the legs are exercised, fitness is built in the legs. If the arms are exercised, fitness is built in the arms. For example, male gymnasts involved only in apparatus events may have good upper body development but poor leg development (13). Finally, the specificity principle applies to certain activities, specificity of training. Specific exercise elicits specific adaptations, creating specific training effects (26). Training is most effective when it closely resembles the activity for which a person is training (13), using the specific muscles involved in the desired performance (32). For example, for an individual to improve the performance of the shot put, the person must perform both an exercise that overloads the arm muscles and a training motion that closely resembles the motion of the shot put (13).

FITNESS FOR LIFE

To maintain a healthy lifestyle, every individual must be fit. You should be physically fit enough so that you can meet the needs of your occupation and daily activities and still be able to enjoy leisure-time activities at the end of a day. By being physically fit, you can gain maximum benefits from your body. As John F. Kennedy said, "Physical fitness is not only one of the most important keys to a healthy body, it is also the basis of dynamic and creative activity."

Why not start now to make your fitness and health a lifetime concern? Physical movement is stimulating and refreshing. There are many types of and variations to exercise programs; you should select one that meets your personal interests and needs. The most important decision, however, is to choose to exercise regularly, *for life*. This book should motivate you to enjoy the fun of exercise through aerobic dance. Wait no longer—read on to see how you can start hopping, running, jumping, and toe touching your way to fitness.

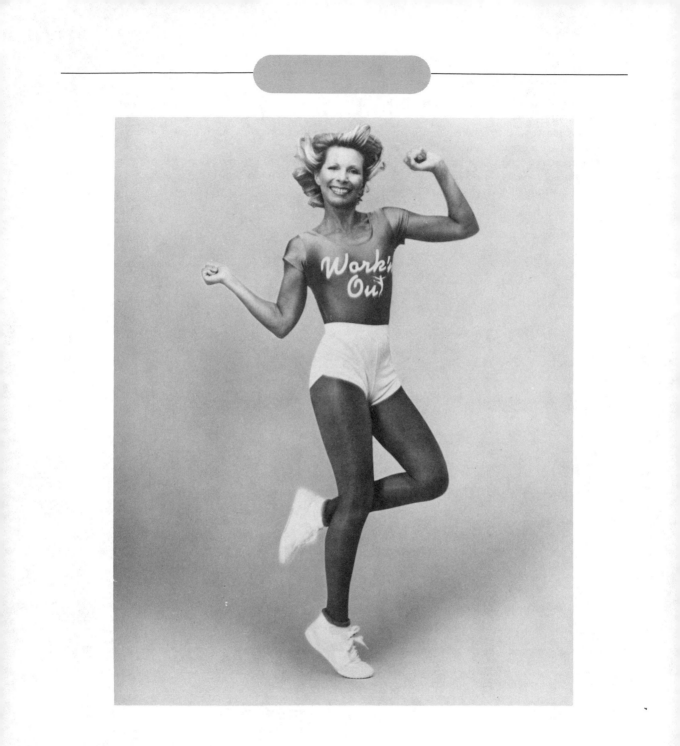

Jacki Sorensen, founder and creator of Aerobic Dance.

Why the Aerobic Workout Is So Important

Chapter

2

Cardiorespiratory fitness is the most important element of physical fitness because it enables the cardiorespiratory system to carry on its functions efficiently under conditions of heavy work and physical stress. An efficient cardiorespiratory system is able to deliver large amounts of oxygen-rich blood to the working muscles over extended periods of time. The format of an aerobic dance class is designed to increase the efficiency of the heart and lungs by incorporating nonstop rhythmic exercises that demand large amounts of oxygen. Thus, regular participation in an aerobic dance class is one of the best ways to improve your cardiorespiratory system.

BODILY CHANGES DURING A WORKOUT

To fully appreciate the value of an aerobic conditioning program, you should understand what happens to your body during the aerobic dance class and the importance and benefits of the workout. The obvious bodily changes that occur during a workout are sweating, heavy breathing, and fatigued muscles. The internal effects from aerobic exercise are not visibly apparent; the heart, lungs, blood vessels, and the body's metabolism all undergo changes.

Heart

During an aerobic workout, both the rate at which the heart beats (heart rate) and the amount of blood the heart pumps per beat (stroke volume) increase so that the total amount of blood the heart pumps in 1 minute (cardiac output) increases. Blood pressure is also affected by aerobic exercise. Systolic blood pressure, a measure of the rhythmic contraction of the heart as blood *leaves* the heart via the ventricles, increases with increased cardiac output. Diastolic blood pressure, a measure of the dilation of the heart cavities while the cavities are *filled* with blood, usually remains the same or slightly decreases (26, 30, 32).

Lungs

During aerobic exercise the body demands more oxygen, so the lungs must deliver more oxygen to the working muscles through the blood. In turn, excess carbon dioxide must be removed from the muscles through the blood. For this accelerated exchange of oxygen and carbon dioxide between the lungs and the blood to occur, both the rate and the depth of breathing must increase (30).

Blood Vessels

During aerobic exercise, the blood vessels shift the blood flow from the visceral (abdominal) organs to the working muscles and to the skin. Thus, those muscles of the body directly involved in exercise and the skin receive more blood, which helps regulate body temperature.

Metabolism

Metabolism is the body's process of converting food into energy through numerous chemical reactions (26). During an aerobic dance workout, as the muscles' need for oxygen increases, more energy is expended, which increases the metabolic rate (how rapidly the body is using its energy stores). Increased metabolic rate allows the body to use more energy, represented by calories, both during the workout and for approximately 1 to 2 hours after the workout.

THE BENEFITS OF AEROBICS

As you become regularly involved in an aerobic dance program, you can look forward to experiencing many of the benefits that accompany aerobic training. Note, however, that each individual will respond differently to the effect of the workout.

Cardiovascular and Respiratory Changes

The muscular strength of the heart increases with aerobic training; the walls of the heart thicken (*hypertrophy*) (30, 32). Stroke volume also increases through aerobic training because the heart has become stronger and is able to eject more blood with each beat. The resting heart rate and the exercise heart rate decrease during aerobic training (32).

With aerobic training, blood volume and hemoglobin increase, facilitating the delivery of oxygen (32). The exercising muscles' ability to extract and use oxygen from the blood improves with regular aerobic exercise (32). As the depth of breathing increases during aerobic exercise, the respiratory muscles must perform additional work and so become more toned. Finally, the amount of breathing needed to perform aerobic exercise decreases, and there is a slight decline in the rate and depth of breathing at rest.

Metabolic Changes

Trained muscles oxidize relatively more fat than do untrained muscles. The mechanism responsible for this change in energy metabolism is not entirely understood, but it may involve a greater capacity of the fat-burning enzymes in trained muscles to oxidize fatty acids (32). With the body's increased ability to metabolize fat there is an increase in the carbohydrate reserve. A conservation of carbohydrates can extend your performance time and let you exercise longer and harder before you become exhausted (30).

Body Composition

Aerobic exercise helps decrease body fat because with increased activity the body derives its energy from its fat stores. Regular participation in an aerobic training program generally reduces total body mass and fat weight; lean body weight may remain constant or increase (2).

Cardiac Risk Changes

Although much scientific evidence supports the view that exercise improves our health and that people who exercise are less susceptible to coronary heart disease, the evidence is still inconclusive. Regular exercise may help prevent the early onset of coronary heart disease (the obstruction of one or more arteries that supply oxygen to the heart), and it may provide a better chance of surviving a heart attack. Until more evidence is available, though, exercise cannot conclusively be prescribed as a preventative for cardiac disease.

Psychological Benefits

For centuries, philosophers have discoursed about the concept of the total person: an individual who has a balanced relationship between mind and body. Health professionals advocate that involvement in regular physical exercise enhances the psychological well-being of a participant by reducing tension and stress, improving sleep habits, and increasing self-esteem and feelings of vitality. Unfortunately, there is not enough scientific evidence to support these beliefs in psychological benefits. However, one premise does remain true: People involved in a regular aerobics exercise program generally feel much better.

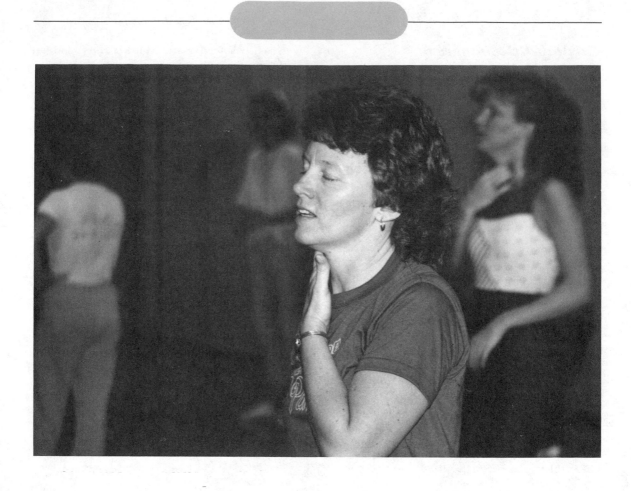

What the Heart Rate Tells Us

Chapter

The heart rate is the most readily obtainable measure of cardiovascular response to exercise. Because the heart rate is directly proportional to the intensity of exercise performed, it tells us whether we are working too hard or not hard enough. The pulse indicates the heartbeat and is counted in beats per minute. You can take your pulse at several different points on your body: the carotid artery in your neck (on each side of your voice box), the radial artery (at the base of your thumb on either arm), or at the temple in front of your ear.

When monitoring your pulse, apply light pressure against the spot, using your index and middle fingers. Never use your thumb when monitoring your pulse because it has a pulse of its own and can give an inaccurate count. With practice, you will get a consistently reliable measure. In an aerobic dance program, it is important to know your rest-

ing heart rate and how to calculate your maximum, target, and recovery heart rates.

RESTING HEART RATE

You should take your resting heart rate (RHR) when you first awake in the morning. At this time, only basal metabolic demands have been made upon the heart, and external stimuli have had no opportunity to affect the resting heart rate. In a comfortable, lying-down position, monitor your pulse for either 6 seconds (multiply the count by 10 to determine pulse rate for 1 minute) or 10 seconds (multiply the count by 6 to determine pulse rate for 1 minute). Typically, after a period of 6 to 8 weeks of aerobic exercise training, the resting heart rate will be lowered (17). Medical textbooks state that the average RHR is 72 beats per minute. Highly trained athletes may have an RHR of

Track Your Resting Heart Rate

N A M E _____

Procedure: Determine your resting heart rate for 60 seconds when you first wake up after a full sleep. Use your first two fingers at the base of your thumb on either arm, at the carotid artery in your neck, on either side of your voice box, at your radial artery, or at your temple.

Initial Assessment

Resting pulse _____   Date _____

8-Week Assessment

Resting pulse _____   Date _____

16-Week Assessment

Resting pulse _____   Date _____

40 beats per minute. The slower resting heart rate means that the heart does not have to beat as often to supply the body with blood and the heart has more rest between beats. You should monitor your RHR after the first 8 weeks of training to evaluate any changes in your heart rate. Use the chart on the facing page to record your resting heart rate over a 16-week period.

Although regular aerobic training programs can reduce the resting heart rate, the following factors can also affect the RHR:

Age: Resting heart rate generally increases with age.

Sex: Resting heart rate is generally higher in women.

Athletic training: Highly trained athletes usually have a lower resting heart rate.

Heredity: If there is a history of low or high resting heart rates within your family, you may inherit that trait.

Emotional stress: Intense emotional states can increase heart rate.

Body temperature: When the body temperature is lower, the heart rate is lower. As the body temperature rises, heart rate increases.

Smoking: Smoking even one cigarette increases the heart rate.

Caffeine: Caffeine intake increases the heart rate.

Physical illnesses: Colds, flu, etc. increase the heart rate.

TARGET OR EXERCISE HEART RATE

When you are exercising to achieve a training effect, your heart must work hard enough to affect your aerobic capacity, but not so hard that you become fatigued. You should attempt to exercise *not* at your maximum heart rate, which is the highest heart rate you can attain and one that is impossible and even dangerous to sustain, but at your target or exercise heart rate.

However, you do need to know your maximum heart rate so you can determine your exercise or target heart rate. You can predict your maximum heart rate by using this formula (20):

Maximum heart rate = 220 − your age

This predicted value varies among people of the same age group. However, the value is accurate enough for estimating your exercise or target heart rate.

Most experts agree that for positive changes to occur in the cardiovascular system, exercise must be performed at an intensity high enough to increase the heart rate to about 70 percent of its maximum. Although no definite evidence is available, the upper limit for training intensity is thought to be about 85 percent of the maximum. For people in relatively poor condition, the training threshold may be closer to 60 percent of their maximum heart rate (32). The upper and lower limits depend a great deal on an individual's initial capacity and state of training.

In 1957, M. J. Karvonen, a Finnish researcher, found from a study of young men that for appreciable gains in cardiorespiratory fitness to occur, during exercise the heart rate must be raised by approximately 60 percent of the difference between the maximum heart rate and the resting heart rate (32):

Exercise heart rate = resting heart rate
+ .60(maximum heart rate − resting heart rate)

Since Karvonen's findings, an increase in heart rate equal to between 70 and 85 percent of the maximum heart rate has been established as a safe and reasonable intensity. Two examples of how to calculate target or exercise heart rate with Karvonen's formula appear on the next page.

It is important that you check your heart rate at various intervals during the aerobic workout. Since heart rate reflects the level of stress on the body, as long as you stay within the bounds of your target zone, you will be exercising safely. Beginners should continually check their pulse so that they do not exceed the high limits of the target zone; exceeding the upper limits brings on early fatigue and could discourage future aerobic activity by causing early burnout.

As the aerobic capacity of your cardiovascular system increases, work will become easier. You will therefore have to increase the intensity of your activities to work at the appropriate target heart rate.

Method	Example 1	Example 2
	A person age 20, with a resting heart rate (RHR) of 80 beats per minute	A person age 40, with a resting heart rate (RHR) of 80 beats per minute

STEP 1

Estimate your maximum heart rate by subtracting your age from 220.	220 − 20 yr 200 maximum heart rate	220 − 40 yr 180 maximum heart rate

STEP 2

Subtract your resting heart rate from your maximum heart rate.	200 max. heart rate − 80 RHR 120	180 max. heart rate − 80 RHR 100

STEP 3

Multiply the answer from step 2 by .6.	$120 \times .6 = 72$	$100 \times .6 = 60$
Multiply the answer from step 2 by .85	$120 \times .85 = 102$	$100 \times .85 = 85$

STEP 4

To each figure in step 3, add your resting heart rate.	$72 + 80 = 152$ $102 + 80 = 182$	$60 + 80 = 140$ $85 + 80 = 165$

STEP 5

The range between these two sums is your target training zone to use while exercising.	Target training zone = 152−182 beats per minute	Target training zone = 140−165 beats per minute

RECOVERY HEART RATE

Your recovery heart rate, which you should take 1 minute after you stop exercising, indicates how quickly you have recovered from the exercise session. Physically fit persons generally recover more rapidly because their cardiovascular systems are more efficient and adapt more quickly to the imposed demands.

The recovery heart rate really has two decreasing phases: the first minute after exercise, during which the heart rate drops sharply, and the *resting plateau,* during which the heart rate gradually decreases. The resting plateau may last as much as 1 hour after exercise. Five minutes following exercise, the heart rate should not exceed 120 beats per minute. After 10 minutes, the heart rate should be below 100 beats per minute. The heart rate should return to its preexercise rate approximately 30 minutes after the exercise session. However, the initial sharp drop in the heart rate that occurs 1 minute after the exercise is the most meaningful indicator of fitness. To determine your rate of recovery, use the following formula:

Recovery heart rate = (exercise heart rate − recovery heart rate after 1 min) ÷ 10

Monitor your exercise pulse immediately at the end of your workout. Exactly 1 minute after the exercise, take your pulse again. Subtract the 1-minute recovery rate from the exercise heart rate and divide this figure by 10. The higher the number for the recovery rate, the more quickly your heart has recovered from the exercise.

Use the following table to evaluate your recovery rate:

Number	Condition
Less than 2	Poor
2 to 3	Fair
3 to 4	Good
4 to 6	Excellent
Above 6	Outstanding

The recovery heart rate also measures the intensity of the workout. Very little drop in the 1-minute pulse indicates that you were probably working too hard and your body is having a difficult time recuperating.

Your heart rate is your best indicator for determining your proper exercise intensity. Take your pulse often throughout the workout, until you learn what your body needs to sustain your target heart rate. Remember—increase the intensity of your exercise if you are not yet in your target range; decrease the intensity if the target rate is too high. Monitor your resting heart rate periodically to evaluate the effects of your aerobic training program. Generally, a lower resting heart rate means a healthier heart.

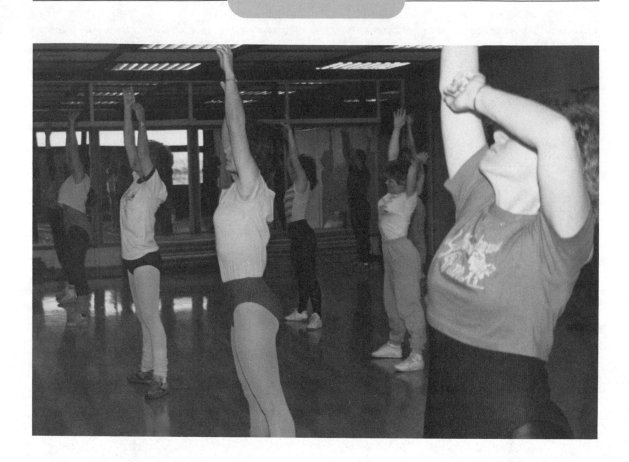

What to Expect in an Aerobic Dance Class

Chapter

The aerobic dance class is a successful combination of exercise, fitness, and fun. If you are enrolling in an aerobic dance class for the first time, you need to know what to expect from the class and what is expected of you in the class. This chapter describes the basic structure of an aerobic dance class and outlines the importance of regular attendance and participation, the need for individualized pacing, and what to wear.

MEDICAL CONSIDERATIONS

Before embarking upon an aerobic dance program, you may want to consider a medical evaluation of your current health status. If you have been following a regular exercise program, an aerobic dance class should pose no physical problems.

However, if you have a serious medical problem and are concerned about the possible effects of increased physical activity, check with your doctor. Your doctor will help you decide whether or not you can safely participate in an aerobic dance class. Students should complete the chart on the next page for the instructor's use.

Aerobic dance combines walking and jogging with jumps, hops, kicks, and lunges as well as basic calisthenics, to improve muscular strength, endurance, and flexibility. Aerobic dance also develops coordination and rhythm by combining simple dance movements into choreographed routines. The routines should be fun and easy to perform with a variety of musical selections. Although all instructors have their own personal lesson formats, the following structure is typical of an aerobic dance class.

Aerobic Student Health History

N A M E _____   A G E _____   D A T E _____

C L A S S _____   S E C T I O N _____

1. Do you have any of the following conditions?

    _____ Diabetes   _____ Epilepsy

    _____ Hypertension   _____ Asthma

2. Have you had any of the following within the past 2 years?

    _____ Heart attack

    _____ Stroke

    _____ Heart surgery

    _____ General major surgery   Please specify _____

3. Do you smoke? Yes _____   No _____

    Cigarettes per day _____   Cigars _____   Pipe _____

4. Are you currently taking any medication? Yes _____   No _____

    If so, please specify _____

5. Are you currently under a doctor's care? Yes _____   No _____

    Reason _____

6. Do you have any handicaps or current injuries that limit your physical

    activity? Yes _____   No _____

    Please specify _____

    _____

7. Date of last physical examination _____

8. According to your physician, are you

    _____ Overweight

    _____ Underweight

    If so, by how much? _____

9. Additional information _____

    _____

WARM-UP

The warm-up warms the body and eases the bodily transition from a resting to a moving state. The warm-up should increase the heart rate and body temperature. In aerobic dance, the warm-up is generally 5 to 10 minutes long and consists of a series of simple stretches for bending, twisting, arching, and curving the spine; stretches for the Achilles tendon, calf muscles, hamstrings, and quadriceps; and loosening exercises for the neck, shoulders, and ankles.

AEROBIC DANCE ROUTINES

Following the warm-up, the aerobic conditioning phase of the lesson begins with aerobic dance routines that vary in length from 12 to 30 minutes. The routines incorporate a myriad of movements that are designed to use all parts of the body and to keep the heart rate at its target zone. The main emphasis is to *keep moving.* Between dances, the pulse rate is often monitored, but even when monitoring your pulse you should maintain at least a walking pace.

BODY TONING EXERCISES

Body toning exercises may follow either the warm-up or the aerobic routines. This exercise period lasts 5 to 20 minutes and stresses muscular strength and flexibility. The exercises concentrate on strengthening and toning the muscles of the arms, abdomen, buttocks, and thighs, with attention to proper body alignment and good exercise technique.

COOL-DOWN

The warm-up prepares the body for activity; the cool-down prepares the body for rest. The cool-down is a series of slow stretches and movements that improve flexibility and gradually slow down the body so that the exercise period does not end abruptly. The exercise tapers from a jog to a walk to the final slow stretches. The cool-down lasts 5 to 10 minutes.

RELAXATION

Rest is the relaxation phase of the exercise cycle. Being able to relax is as important to the body as being able to successfully withstand imposed physical demands. The relaxation phase of the aerobic dance lesson is 5 to 10 minutes long.

Throughout the lesson, the instructor gives the whole class instructions on the technique for certain exercises. The instructor should offer individual students constructive criticism.

REGULAR ATTENDANCE

To achieve fitness benefits from an aerobic dance program, you must attend class (or participate in aerobic activity) at least three times a week for a minimum of 20 minutes. These classes should be evenly distributed throughout the week, with a maximum of two days' rest between classes. If you must miss a class, substitute a jog, quick walk, or another aerobic activity within the week.

If you are ill or unable to exercise over a certain length of time, it is important to gradually work your way back to your former level of activity. It may take you three or more classes after an illness to perform with the same energy you expended prior to your absence. With regular participation, you can maintain and improve fitness levels.

INDIVIDUAL PACE

We have all heard the fitness axioms "Train, don't strain" and "No pain, no gain." Somewhere between these two ideas is a middle ground that provides the safest and most productive workout pace. You are not competing with anyone but yourself in aerobic dance, so it is important to work at your own level; set the pace that is most beneficial for your own body. Keep breathing easily, and never hold your breath. If you can carry on a conversation when performing aerobic dance, you are working at the correct pace.

In aerobic dance, the heartbeat is regularly monitored to help establish a pace that will push a person to achieve but not overexert. Aerobic dance routines are choreographed so that, depending upon the individual fitness level, sections of routines allow students to walk, jog, or run.

WHAT TO WEAR

Comfortable clothing that allows ease of movement is appropriate attire for aerobic dancing. Sweatsuits and jogging apparel provide layers that you can remove as your body temperature increases. Once your body is warm, simple jogging shorts and a T-shirt or dance leotard and tights are sufficient. Cotton is the best material for exercise wear because it absorbs perspiration. As cotton becomes damp, the air evaporates the moisture and cools your body.

The fashion industry has provided an assortment of specialty aerobic dance apparel. Overgarments that superficially heat the body include legwarmers; wool unitards and tights; nylon rip pants, shorts, and tops. These clothing items should be worn only as overgarments or to warm up the body. A popular notion is that use of these items during a workout can lead to quick weight loss, but in truth you are only sweating off water—not fat! In warm weather you should wear the minimum amount of clothing so you can sweat freely and let your cooling system work.

Support undergarments are important apparel in aerobic dance. Women should wear a bra that fits snugly and provides adequate support during the vigorous running and jumping movements in class. Men should wear athletic supporters or dance belts for adequate support during exercise activities.

Shoes are the major monetary investment for an aerobic dance class. Well-constructed and well-fitting shoes are necessary for working on hard surfaces, so make sure when you test the shoe that you do not just move on a carpeted surface. Find a hard surface in the store or request permission to test the shoe outdoors. Shoes are not only for comfort but for helping to prevent injuries such as shin splints, heel bruises, straining of the Achilles tendon, and blisters. The following guidelines will help you select proper shoes for aerobic dance:

1. A shoe should be designed to absorb the repeated stress the knees, calves, and ankles receive. The arch and heel should have several layers of cushioning to absorb the shock of

the foot continually landing on the ground. Good cushioning under the ball of the foot is also important.

2. Select a shoe that will support lateral movements. A shoe with a wide heel flair restricts lateral movement and is more appropriate for the forward movement of jogging.

3. Shoes with nylon uppers are cooler for the foot, require less care, and are lighter than shoes with leather uppers.

4. The fit of the shoe is extremely important. The heel should fit snugly. The front of the shoe should be wide enough to accommodate the foot; there should be plenty of room for the toes to move comfortably inside the shoe. When fitting the shoe, take the time to walk, jog, and jump to test the "feel" of the shoe.

Many shoe companies presently make shoes specifically designed for aerobic dance. Any shoes that meet the four guidelines are appropriate for class. An athletic shoe store has the largest and best selection of shoes. Wear cotton socks with shoes to keep your feet dry and free of blisters. Use foot powder or foot spray if your feet perspire heavily.

(Besides proper footwear for preventing injury, the composition of the dance floor is extremely important and should be investigated when you are choosing a class. Cement covered with carpet is the worst flooring because it gives the illusion of being cushioned, yet cement is the hardest possible surface. Hardwood flooring is the best surface for aerobic dance.)

WHAT TO BRING TO CLASS

A few additional items may be useful in your aerobic dance class: floor mat, towel, sweatbands, and light weights.

Floor Mat

A mat provides padded support for your body as you do floor exercises. If mats are not available at the class, you can buy a lightweight mat at most athletic stores, in the athletic department at a major department store, or at a chain drugstore. Any mat that is easy to carry and has some padding is sufficient.

Towel

A towel is useful in class if you perspire heavily. You can also use a towel to cover your mat, which is especially advisable if the mat is plastic because the towel will help absorb the additional perspiration the plastic creates.

Sweatbands

If you do not have a towel, wear a sweatband around your head and wrists to collect perspiration. Elasticized cotton sweatbands are easy to slip on and off. You can also use a bandana rolled and tied around your head as a sweatband.

Light Weights

When exercising your arms and legs, you may want to use light weights to apply an overload to these body parts. You can buy two kinds of light weights. One type normally fastens with Velcro around the ankles and wrists; another type is made specifically for the arms and is hand-held.

CHECKLIST FOR A MORE SUCCESSFUL CLASS

1. Arrive at class 10 to 15 minutes early to give yourself time for pre-warm-up exercises.
2. Do not eat a heavy meal prior to class. Fruit, yogurt, dried fruit, or nuts are recommended preclass snacks.
3. Come to class in the appropriate dance attire.
4. Clear your mind of outside interference when you enter the classroom. Be prepared to fully concentrate on the lesson.
5. Find a space to stand where you can see and hear the teacher. Allow yourself plenty of room so you can move and stretch freely.
6. Be sensitive to any injuries you might have. Pay special attention to the injured area during pre-warm-up exercises as well as class activities.
7. Work at your correct heart rate so you can keep moving and get maximum benefits from the workout.
8. Do not compare yourself to others in the class. Listen to your body!
9. Do not be afraid to ask questions if you are unclear about a step or exercise.
10. Bring a container of water for an occasional drink to avoid dehydration.
11. Participate in aerobic dance to improve your fitness, your posture, your knowledge of your body, and to have a good time!

Now that you know what to expect in your aerobic dance class, it is time to get started. The last ingredients to bring to class are the enthusiasm for doing your best and the attitude that you will have a good time!

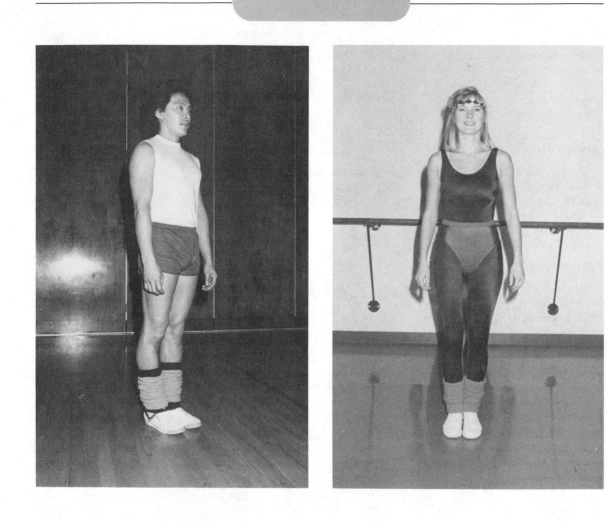

Posture Perfect—or Imperfect?

Chapter

5

There are several reasons why the aerobic dancer needs good posture: Good posture is the basis for effective movement patterns, it helps prevent injury, and aesthetically it creates the best body image. Correct skeletal alignment is also necessary, to establish maximum balance and ease of movement. This chapter describes correct posture and body alignment and presents exercises to help you achieve correct posture.

DEFINITIONS OF POSTURE AND ALIGNMENT

Posture is the position of the body or the body's bearing or carriage. *Alignment,* as used in aerobic dance, is the relationship of the body segments to each other. When the body is in correct vertical alignment, there is minimum strain on the muscles and ligaments attached to the weight-bearing joints.

Correct alignment depends on a balanced relationship between the front (anterior) and the back (posterior) postural muscles (see Figure 5-1). Most of the largest muscles in the body are involved with the body's maintenance of correct alignment. These muscles are classified as the anteroposterior antigravity muscles and are identified in Figure 5-1. The antigravity musculature helps the body adequately resist the pull of gravity so it can maintain an erect posture. These muscles must be well conditioned to withstand the stresses gravity imposes and to resist the skeletal framework's tendency to collapse with the force of gravity.

The downward pressure of gravity tends to make the skeletal framework misalign at three principal areas: the ankles, knees, and hips. To counteract this effect, the anteroposterior muscles must maintain a muscular tension balance. The muscles that maintain lower limb balance are the gastrocnemius

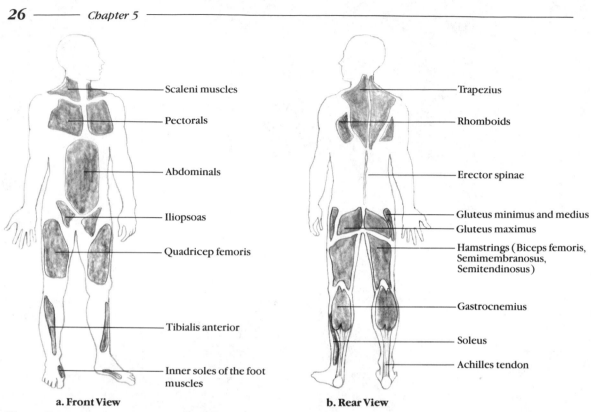

a. Front View

b. Rear View

Figure 5-1 *General location of postural muscles.*

and soleus at the ankle, the quadriceps femoris at the knee, and the gluteus maximus at the hip. The trunk is held erect by the erector spinae muscles running from the base of the skull to the sacrum. To balance the trunk's posterior aspect, the abdominals maintain the proper relationship between the ribcage and pelvis on the body's anterior aspect (19). An unbalanced relationship among these muscles will cause postural deviations.

ALIGNMENT REFERENCE POINTS

Every individual's body structure has minor variations, but there are visual guidelines for evaluating correct alignment. In a side view of correct alignment, an imaginary line of gravity passes through the following body reference points (see Figure 5-2):

Front of the ankle bone
Back of the kneecap
Center of the hip
Middle of the shoulder
Behind the top of the ear

In a back view of correct alignment, the imaginary line of gravity passes through the following body reference points (see Figure 5-3):

Midway between the heels
Through the cleft of the buttocks
Through the midpoint of all vertebrae
Through the center of the head

PLACEMENT

Placement, as used in aerobic dance, is the relative positioning of the separate body parts so that

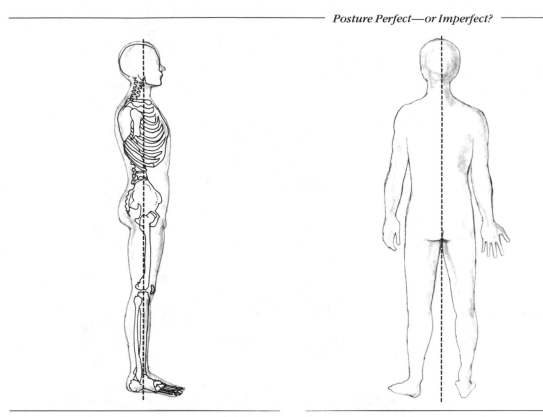

Figure 5-2 *Line of gravity, side view.*   **Figure 5-3** *Line of gravity, back view.*

the body can be in total and correct alignment (see Figures 5-2 and 5-3). You should become familiar with the proper placement of the major body parts—head and neck, shoulder girdle, ribcage, pelvis, knees, and feet—and use a mirror to go through a mental checklist of their proper placement in all positions and movements. With practice, you will develop a kinesthetic awareness of proper placement and will not have to use a mirror; eventually, proper placement will become second nature to you.

Head and Neck

The head, the heaviest body segment, rests on the neck, which is a small flexible segment. The head should be carried directly atop the neck, protruding neither forward nor backward. There should be a sense of the neck stretching away from the spine so that both the back and the front of the neck are long. With the head and neck in correct alignment, a vertical line can be drawn from the top of the ear to the middle of the shoulder. The first alignment exercise will enable you to experience the proper placement of the head and neck.

Shoulder Girdle

The shoulder girdle—consisting of the collarbones in front and the shoulder blades in back—should be placed directly above the ribcage. The shoulder girdle is attached to the trunk only at the sternum (breastbone), allowing it to move freely. The shoulders should not be pulled back or allowed to slump forward; they should point directly to the side, so that the chest and the shoulder blades are equally open. The arms should hang freely in the shoulder sockets. The shoulders should be lowered and the neck lengthened to increase the distance between the shoulders and the ears. The second and third alignment exercises will enable you to experience the proper placement of the shoulder girdle.

Ribcage

The ribcage floats above the pelvis and is connected in back to the spinal column. The ribcage should be lifted upward from the pelvis to create a long-waisted appearance. Do not hyperextend the ribcage. The fourth alignment exercise will enable you to experience the proper placement of the ribcage.

Pelvis

The pelvis is the keystone of the skeleton. The tilt of the pelvis affects the posture of the entire body and the distribution of the body's weight over the feet. To be correctly placed, the pelvis should be in a centered position, which lengthens the lumbar spine and shortens the abdominal muscles. Extreme forward or backward tilting of the pelvis can injure the lumbar spine and muscles of the lower back. The fifth and sixth alignment exercises will enable you to experience the proper placement of the pelvis.

Knees

The position of the knees is affected by the placement of the pelvis; the knees should be directly above and in line with the direction of the toes. In the standing position, the knees should be slightly relaxed. *Hyperextension* (knees locked or pressed too far back) is a common error.

Feet

The pelvis is the keystone of the skeletal structure; the feet are the main base of support. In a static position, the greatest support is achieved when the weight of the body is equally distributed over the metatarsal arch (the ball of the foot), the base of the big toe, the base of the small toe, and the heel (see Figure 5-4). All the toes should remain in contact with the floor, to provide the widest pos-

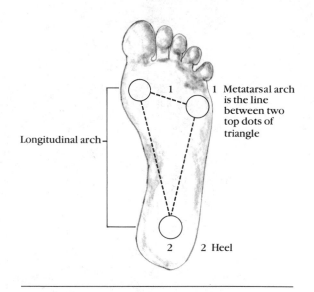

Figure 5-4 *Weight-bearing areas in the foot.*

sible base of support. In addition, the longitudinal arch should be well lifted to prevent the ankle from rolling inward.

EXERCISES FOR ACHIEVING GOOD ALIGNMENT

The following exercises will help you achieve correct body alignment. They can easily be performed in 10 minutes. We recommend that you perform them daily until correct alignment becomes a habit.

Starting position for exercises: Lie on your back, with your knees bent, the soles of your feet flat on the ground, your arms by the side of your body, and the palms of both your hands flat on the floor.

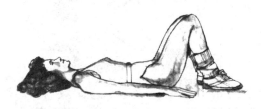

Starting position

PLACEMENT OF HEAD AND NECK

Assume the starting position with your hands clasped behind your head (not your neck). Lift your head only off the floor and pull your elbows together. You should feel a stretch at the base of your neck and all down your spine. Slowly place your head back on the floor, stretching your neck away from your spine. Repeat this stretch three times. Maintain this lengthened neck alignment throughout the remaining exercises.

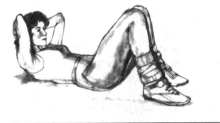

Placement of head and neck

PLACEMENT OF SHOULDER GIRDLE

Assume the starting position and then place both your hands on your hipbones. Keeping your elbows in contact with the floor, use an isometric (static) stretch to point your elbows toward the sides of the room. Hold the position for 10 seconds and then relax. Repeat this stretch four times. Although the movement of this exercise is slight, when executed properly it equally expands the back and chest. Maintain this back and chest expansion throughout the remaining exercises.

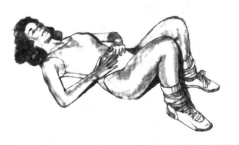

Shoulder girdle alignment: Elbows touching floor

PLACEMENT OF SHOULDER GIRDLE

Assume the starting position, with your hands placed on your hipbones. Isolate your shoulders by lifting them forward off the floor. Hold this position for 5 seconds. Relax and place your shoulders in total contact with the floor. As you perform this exercise, try to create the greatest distance possible between your shoulders and ears, to help maintain the correct shoulder and neck alignment. Repeat the exercise four times.

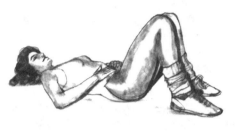

Shoulder girdle alignment: Shoulders lifted off and then returned to floor

PLACEMENT OF RIBCAGE

Assume the starting position, with your hands on your hipbones. Lift your ribcage forward off the floor, to create an extreme arch in your back. Reverse the action, pressing your ribcage back against the floor, or farther toward the spine. Repeat the exercise four times, ending with your ribcage in its correct placement against the floor.

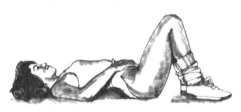

Placement of ribcage

PLACEMENT OF PELVIS

Assume the starting position, with your arms stretched on the floor over your head, and take

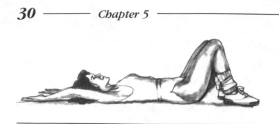

Pelvis alignment: Arms above head

deep breaths. As you exhale, contract your abdominal muscles so that your lower back is in total contact with the floor. Hold this position, concentrating on the position of your lower back and stomach. Repeat the exercise four times.

PLACEMENT OF PELVIS

Assume the starting position and maintain the alignment of your lower back as in the exercise for the placement of head and neck. Slowly stretch your arms on the floor above your head; hold the

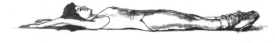

Pelvis alignment: Arms above head, legs stretched out

stretched position several seconds, keeping your lower back against the floor. Relax and release your back to allow the natural curve of your spine to return. With your arms in the stretched position, straighten your legs along the floor, without locking your knees. Hold this position for several seconds, keeping your lower back against the floor. Return to the starting position. Repeat the exercise four times.

Mentally review the correct alignment of the body parts:

1. Lower back in contact with the floor
2. Abdominal muscles contracted
3. Back and chest open and equally expanded, with elbows pointing to the side
4. Neck and ears stretching away from the spine and shoulders
5. Shoulders resting flat against the floor
6. Legs straight, without the knees being locked
7. Breathing full and easy

Once you attain the proper body placement on the floor, try to achieve the same posture in the standing position. When you attain correct alignment in the standing position, try to maintain this alignment while walking and performing aerobic dance movements.

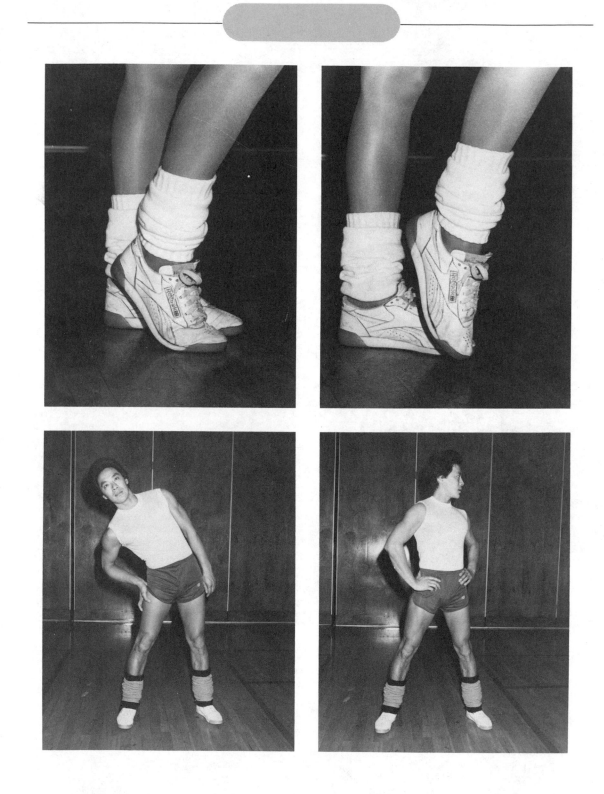

Warm-up

Chapter

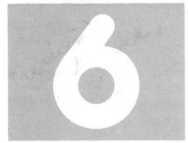

A warm-up is like tuning a fine instrument. The body, the aerobic dancer's instrument, must be tuned in preparation to responding to the demands placed upon it in an aerobic dance workout.

Most professionals highly recommend the warm-up, although there is little scientific evidence that it helps performance or prevents injury. However, the warm-up is recommended for several reasons. First, it is believed that warm-up shortens the cardiovascular and muscular systems' adjustment period to the oncoming stress of physical activity. The warm-up thus lets the body gradually shift from a resting state to an active state without undue shock.

Second, the warm-up is thought to minimize the risk of inadequate blood flow to the heart during the first few seconds of heavy exercise because it gives the heart time to adjust from being at rest to undergoing sudden, strenuous activity (5). The warm-up raises the body's intake of oxygen, which improves the body's biochemical reactions and which in turn is believed to improve physical performance (31).

The warm-up increases the temperature of the muscles, allowing the muscles to more rapidly and forcefully contract and more rapidly relax. This response is thought to improve performance (15). Finally, the warm-up is also thought to be an important psychological benefit because it mentally prepares a person for the strenuous demands of the upcoming workout. Many experts believe that exercise prior to a strenuous activity gradually prepares a person to go all out without fear of injury. In competitive athletics, many competitors consider the warm-up an activity that prepares them mentally for their event, an opportunity for them to clearly focus their concentration or to psyche up for the upcoming performance (32).

WARM-UP CONCEPTS

We believe that a warm-up is valuable before engaging in the vigorous aerobic dance workout. To attain a thorough warm-up, you should adhere to certain concepts. The warm-up is *not* a time for intense stretching; it is a time to loosen and ready the muscles for the aerobic dances to follow. The warm-up should consist of a variety of movements, including exercises involving calisthenics, stretching, and general body movements (32).

To warm up properly, start slowly and gradually increase the pace and intensity of the exercise until your body begins to feel loose and warm. Rhythmic exercises that flow from one sequence to the next help you ease gradually into stretch positions. The time necessary for warm-up varies with each individual, depending upon fitness level and age. Generally, a minimum warm-up of 5 to 10 minutes is adequate. Pre-warm-up exercises can help those who want more warm-up activity. For such individual pre-warm-up, allow yourself approximately 10 minutes before class. Use the simple exercises described in this chapter, and be sure to pay extra attention to warming up any area of your body that is weak or prone to injury.

Exercise stretches should be static rather than ballistic (bouncing). A slow static stretch tends to counteract a muscle's stretch reflex, whereas the sudden stretch of a ballistic exercise contracts the muscle, which negates the purpose of the stretch (19). In addition, static stretching requires less expenditure of energy, which probably causes less muscle soreness and yields more relief from muscular distress (15).

Light perspiration may be an indication that your muscles are warm and ready for more intense exercise. As we mentioned earlier, your body should feel warm and loose, ready for movement. After you complete your warm-up routine, begin your workout immediately so that you will not lose the benefits of the warm-up.

HEAD AND NECK EXERCISES

ISOLATIONS

Move your head up and then down. Tilt your head from side to side. Look to your right and left.

HEAD CIRCLES

Roll your head in a full circle, letting your neck muscles relax but being sure to maintain good posture in the upper body so that your neck muscles get maximum stretch.

———————————————— PRECAUTIONS ————————————

- Do not force your neck to arch or hyperextend. Quick, abrupt moves can damage the ligaments in the neck.
- When doing head circles, avoid rolling your head to the back because this could put unnecessary tension on the cervical vertebrae.

SHOULDER AND CHEST EXERCISES

Starting position for exercises: Stand with your feet shoulder width apart.

SHOULDER CIRCLES

Circle your shoulders forward, up, back, and down, stretching fully. Reverse the directions and gradually increase your speed.

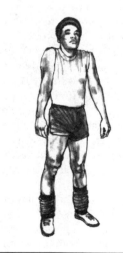

Shoulder circles

SHOULDER SHRUGS

Elevate your shoulders to your ears and then press your shoulders down. Lift both shoulders together and then one shoulder at a time.

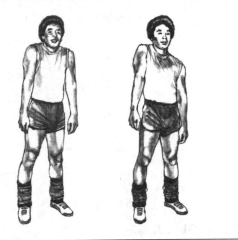

Shoulder shrugs

CHEST STRETCH

Clasp your hands behind your back and stretch your chest muscles by pulling your shoulder blades together. You can also perform the chest stretch while bending forward at your waist and lifting your clasped hands away from your lower back, toward the ceiling.

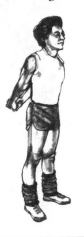

Chest stretch

RIBCAGE AND WAIST EXERCISES

LATERAL STRETCH

Stand with your feet shoulder width apart. Bend *sideways* from your waist. Be sure you do not lean forward or backward; bend directly sideways. Do not move below your waist. To protect your lower back, support your trunk with your hand on your thigh or your forearm on your thigh, keeping your knees slightly bent. For additional leverage, you can stretch your opposite arm overhead.

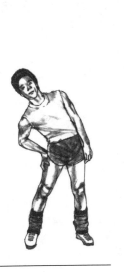
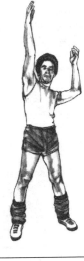

Lateral stretch   *Reach stretch*

REACH STRETCH

Reach up to the ceiling with one arm at a time. Fully stretch your side and ribcage. Do not hyperextend your ribcage or your lower back.

SPINAL TWIST

Stabilize your lower body by standing with your feet slightly apart and your knees slightly bent. Fully twist your upper body above your waist. Your arms can be in a variety of positions. Make sure your knees stay directly over your toes. Twist *gradually,* to avoid placing any possible strain on the spinal ligaments.

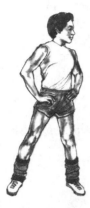

Spinal twist

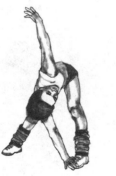

Triangle stretch

TRIANGLE STRETCH

Standing in a wide straddle position, with your knees slightly bent, touch your right hand to your left foot. Stretch your left arm to the ceiling, and twist your upper body so you are looking at your upraised left arm. Hold this position for 10 to 15 seconds and then reverse to the opposite side. If you are a beginner or have tight hamstring muscles, keep one knee flexed at all times.

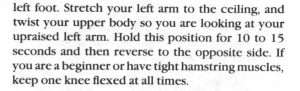

——————————— PRECAUTIONS ———————————

- Before flexing your trunk forward, *always* perform a lateral stretch or spinal twist because these exercises help release tension in the spinal muscles.
- Beginners, until your hamstring and lower back muscles achieve reasonable flexibility, in all forward bending movements keep your knees slightly bent to avoid placing undue stress on one of the main supporting ligaments in the spine: the posterior longitudinal ligament.

HIP AND BUTTOCKS EXERCISES

BENT LEG REACH-THROUGH

Standing in a wide straddle position with your feet parallel, bend your knees and reach through your legs. Relax your neck and head.

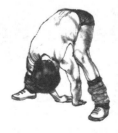

Bent leg reach-through

WIDE AND DEEP KNEE BEND AND STRETCH

Standing in a wide straddle position with your legs turned out from your hip joint, bend deeply at your knees, keeping your heels flat on the ground. Press your thighs open with your elbows. Now straighten your legs and turn your feet into a parallel position, with your hands reaching toward or touching the floor. Do not hyperextend your knees when straightening your legs. Relax your neck and head.

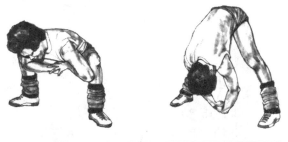

Wide and deep knee bend and stretch

LOOSE SWING

Standing with your feet together and parallel, stretch your arms toward the ceiling and then swing your arms forward and down, releasing your upper body while bending your knees. Return to the starting position by swinging your arms and body upward and straightening your legs. Perform the exercise slowly.

THIGH, HAMSTRING, AND LOWER LEG EXERCISES

RUNNER LUNGE AND STRETCH

This exercise stretches the quadriceps, hamstrings, and the Achilles tendon. From a deep lunge position, with your feet parallel, place your hands on the floor on either side of your forward bent knee. In this position, the heel of your front foot must remain on the floor; your back leg should be straight, with your foot fully flexed and your toes pressed against the floor. Keeping your hands on the floor, straighten your front leg while pressing the heel of your back foot to the floor. Try to keep your back flat, pressing your chest toward your front knee. For additional stretch, flex the foot of your front leg, lifting the toes off the floor. Return to the lunge position and repeat the stretch sequence on your opposite leg.

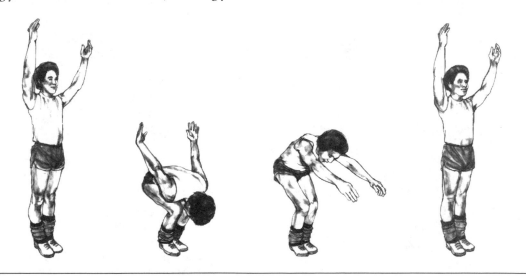

Loose swing

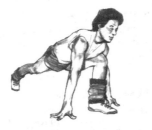

Runner lunge and stretch

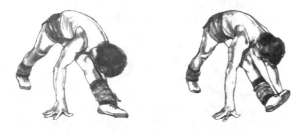

Runner lunge and stretch

PARALLEL FORWARD STRETCH

This exercise stretches the hamstrings. Standing with your feet together and parallel, with your knees slightly bent, bend over and place your hands on or near the floor. Fully bend your knees, letting your heels release from the floor. Try to lift your heels as high off the floor as possible, and stretch your feet in this position. Next, keeping your hands on the floor, return your heels to the floor and try to straighten your legs, remembering to keep your knees slightly bent in the forward stretch position.

Parallel forward stretch

HAND WALK

This exercise stretches the hamstring muscles at the back of the thigh (see Figure 5-1) and the Achilles tendon, which runs from the heel to the back calf muscles. Begin in the parallel forward stretch position, with your feet together and parallel, knees slightly bent, and hands on the floor. Walk your hands as far away from your feet as possible, attempting to keep your heels in contact with the floor. Try to keep your back flat during the hand walk. Hold the stretch 10 seconds and then walk your hands back toward your feet.

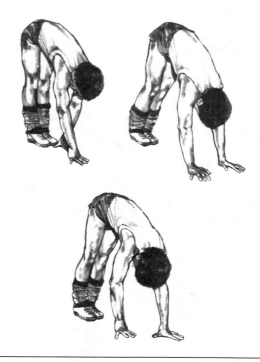

Hand walk

TREADING

In the hand-walk position, with your hands walked away from your feet, bend your right knee, lifting your heel off the floor while the heel of your left straight leg remains in contact with the floor. Reverse the position by lifting your left heel off the floor and pressing your right leg straight and your

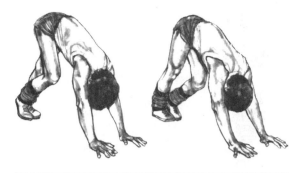

Treading

right heel to the floor. Alternate the treading between your right and left legs until your Achilles tendon feels adequately stretched.

SIDE LUNGE

Standing in a wide straddle position with your legs turned out from your hip joint, lunge by bending one knee and keeping your other leg straight. You can lift the heel of your bent leg or keep it on the floor. If you lift your heel, the stretch will be emphasized on the inner thigh of your straight leg. If you keep the heel on the floor, the stretch will also involve the calf muscles of your bent leg. Make sure you do not compress your knee more than 90°. Your hands can remain on the floor for balance. You can use your arms to help keep your bent knee directly over the direction of your feet and toes.

KNEE LIFT

This exercise stretches the hamstrings. Standing with your feet parallel, pull one knee to your chest by holding your leg underneath the thigh. You can also perform this stretch while lying on the floor with your legs together and fully extended. Pull one knee to your chest, grasping the lower part of your leg with your hands clasped. The leg remaining on the floor must remain straight and fully extended.

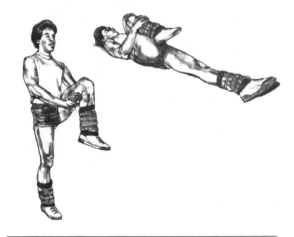

Knee lifts

CALF STRETCH

Start by standing with your feet together and parallel. Step with one foot forward so that your feet are approximately 1 to 2 feet apart. Lunge onto your front leg, being sure to keep your back leg

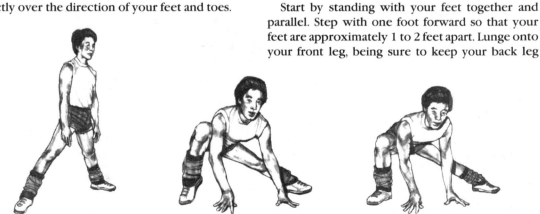

Side lunge

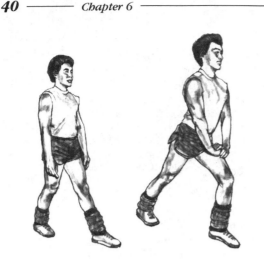

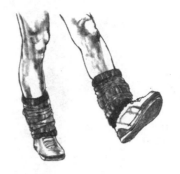

Ankle flexion

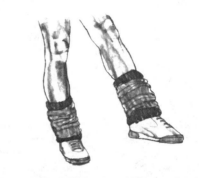

Ankle extension

Calf stretch

straight and your back toes directed forward. Both your heels remain on the floor. Your hands can rest on your front leg as an added weight to stretch your back leg.

PRECAUTIONS

- In all forward bending movements, keep your knees slightly bent to avoid placing undue stress on one of the main supporting spinal ligaments: the posterior longitudinal ligament.
- In all exercises involving bent knees, keep the pressure off your knees by maintaining good body alignment, and keep your knees directly in line with your feet and toes.

ANKLE EXERCISES

ANKLE FLEXION AND EXTENSION

Standing or sitting, flex (point your foot up) and then extend (point your foot down) your ankle slowly.

ANKLE CIRCLES

Standing or sitting, slowly circle your ankle with your foot flexed and then with your foot extended.

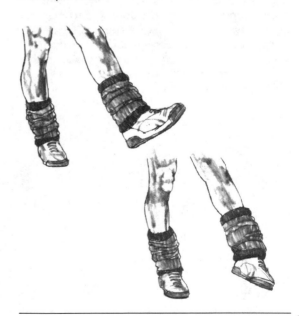

Ankle circles

When flexing or extending your ankles, maintain a straight line from your big toe to your ankle to avoid toeing in and excessively stretching the muscles on the outside of your ankle.

WARM-UP ROUTINES AND PRECAUTIONS

The exercises described can be combined in many ways. For maximum benefit, you must perform repetitions of each exercise. When you are creating routines, it is important that transitions between exercises are smooth and flow naturally. Music for warm-up routines can be any top 40 favorite, as long as it has a steady, rhythmic beat and preferably a 4/4 time signature or one that can be counted in 4 or 8 beats.

Warm-up exercises should begin slowly; gradually increase your effort until you reach moderate pace and intensity. Choose rhythmic movements that flow from one sequence to the next. Keep your hips stable when performing exercises involving a lateral stretch or twisting of the torso. Always perform a lateral stretch or torso twist before flexing your trunk forward. These exercises help release tension in the spinal muscles. Always include exercises for the Achilles tendon and the calf muscles since these body parts are heavily used in aerobic dance. Immediately begin your aerobic workout when you complete your warm-up. Finally and most importantly, remember that the warm-up must do just that—warm you up and prepare you for the vigorous workout ahead!

The following routines work with any song that can be counted in 4 or 8 beats. The musical choice is your own; just be sure it is something that inspires you to move!

Warm-up Routine 1

Exercise	*Repetitions*	*Counts*
Head circles	2 right, 2 left	4 for each circle
Shoulder shrugs	4 times	4 for each shrug
Lateral stretch with both arms reaching	4 times, alternating right and left	4 to reach lateral; 4 to reach center
Flat back	8 times	1 for each flat back
Bent leg reach-through	8 times	1 each
Triangle stretch	4 times, alternating right and left	4 each
Treading	16 times	4 to walk hands out and bring feet together; 2 for each tread
Parallel forward stretch	4 sets	4 to walk hands back; 4 knees bent; 4 legs straight
Roll spine up to vertical position	1 time	8
Calf stretch	2 times, alternating right and left	8 each
Loose swing	4 times	4 each
Open arms and finish with your hands at your sides		8

Chapter 6

Warm-up Routine 2

Exercise	Repetitions	Counts
Reach stretch	8 times	2 each
Spinal twist	8 times alternating right and left	2 each
Chest stretch	1 time	4 to open arms to side; 4 to clasp hands; 8 bending at waist
Parallel forward stretch	2 sets	4 knees bent; 4 legs straight
Roll spine up to vertical position		8
Runner lunge	1 time right and left	8 down; 8 legs straight; 8 foot flexed
Hand walk		4 to walk forward; 8 to hold; 4 to walk back
Side lunge with arm reaching over bent leg	4 times, alternating right and left	4 for each lunge
Knee lift with ankle circle outward and then inward	4 times, alternating right and left	8 for ankle circle outward; 8 for ankle circle inward
Hang over to touch floor		8
Roll spine up to vertical position		8

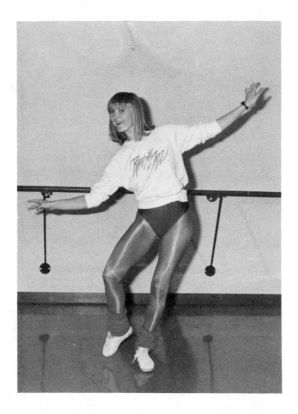

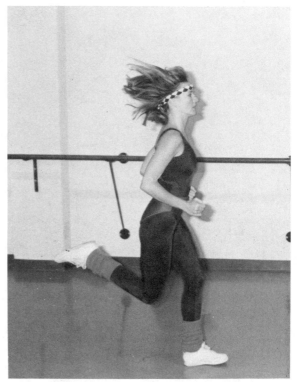

Aerobic Dances

Chapter

Aerobic dances consist of steps and movements drawn from pedestrian locomotor movements that are stylized by the addition of movements from a variety of dance forms, including jazz, ballet, modern, folk, square, and social dance, and performed to music. Aerobic dance movements, done during the aerobic session of the class, must be performed *nonstop* for a minimum of 15 minutes and must sustain an individual's target heart rate. You must pace yourself so that you can complete the entire aerobic section of the workout. If you find yourself tiring, slow down, but *never* come to a complete stop. *Reminder:* Carefully monitor your target heart rate by taking your pulse after the first dance and then periodically throughout the rest of the session.

This chapter describes locomotor movements and dance steps commonly used in aerobic dances, discusses combinations of these movements, and outlines precautions to follow in the aerobic dance class. A discussion of how to choreograph an aerobic dance routine and several examples of such routines are also included.

LOCOMOTOR MOVEMENTS

The basic locomotor movements used in aerobic dance are walking, running, jumping, hopping, leaping, skipping, and sliding. Variations of these movements are created by integrating arm and footwork patterns and directional changes; the variations are then enlivened with snaps, claps, and body slaps.

Walking

A walk is a transfer of weight from one foot to the other, with one foot always on the ground.

Variations

Walking in place
Walking forward
Walking backward
Walking diagonally
Walking in a circle
Turning
Walking on your toes
Walk forward and then step together; walk back-
    ward and then step together; walk sideways
    and then step together
Walking in a Square

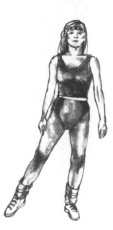

Walking sideways, right foot to side

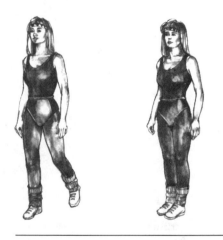

Walking forward, step together

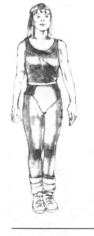

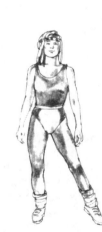

Step together   *Walking sideways, left foot to side*

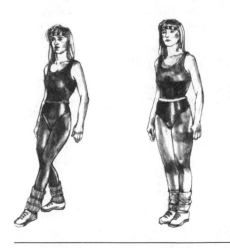

Walking backward, step together

Grapevine
1. Step to the right side with your right foot.
2. Step so your left foot crosses behind your
   right foot.
3. Step to your right side with your right foot.
4. Step so your left foot crosses in front of
   your right foot.

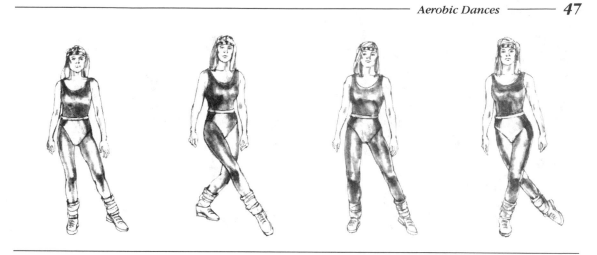

Grapevine

Running

A run is a transfer of weight from one foot to the other. At one point in a run, both feet are off the ground. A run is faster than a walk.

Variations

Running in place
Running forward
Running backward
Running diagonally
Running in a circle
Running in a figure eight
Grapevine
High-knee runs

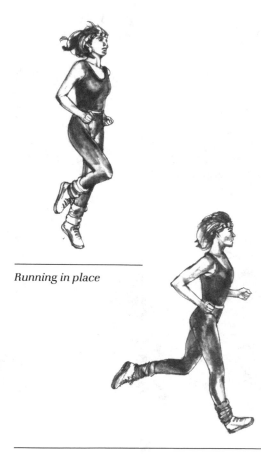

Running in place

—————— PRECAUTIONS ——————

· When running forward, run with your knees lifted and land with your heel first, to put less stress on the calf muscles. Follow through by rolling onto the ball of your foot.
· When running in place, run with your knees lifted and land with the ball of your foot first. Follow through by pressing your heel to the floor.

Running forward

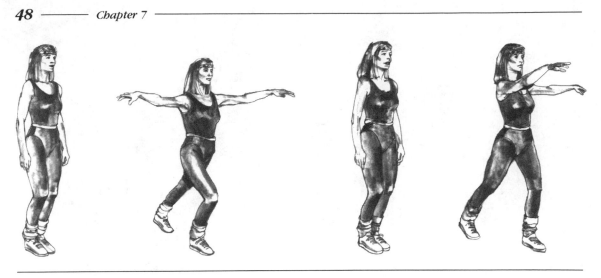

Scissors jumping jacks

Jumping

A jump is an aerial movement in which a person takes off from two feet and lands on two feet.

Variations

Jumping in place
Jumping forward
Jumping backward
Jumping sideward
Jumping diagonally

Quarter, half, and whole turns
Regular jumping jacks
Scissors jumping jacks
1. Jump with your feet together.
2. Jump with your legs splitting front and back.
3. Alternate legs on the split jump.
4. Swing arms in opposition.
Crossover jumping jacks
1. Jump to a straddle position, your feet apart.
2. Jump crossing your legs.

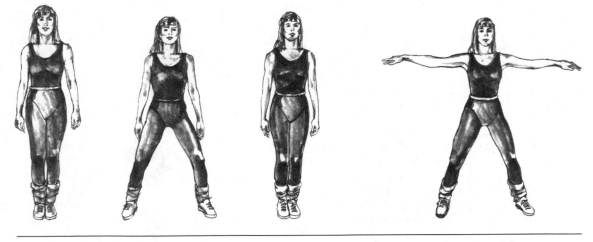

Progressive jumping jacks

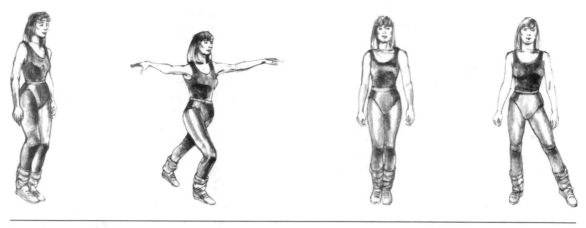

Jump lunge

3. Alternate crossing your legs front and back.
Progressive jumping jacks
    1. Jump in place.
    2. Jump to a straddle position, feet apart.
    3. Jump your feet together.
    4. Jump to a straddle position, feet apart; raise your arms to shoulder height.
    5. Jump feet together and bring your arms down to the side.

    6. Do a regular jumping jack, clapping your hands overhead.
    7. Jump feet together and bring your arms down to the side.
    8. Perform the sequence in reverse order.

Jump lunge: Alternately jump in place and then jump to a lunge position forward, backward, and sideways.

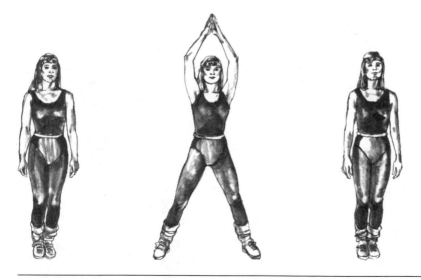

Progressive jumping jacks (continued)

Hopping

A hop is an aerial movement in which a person takes off on one foot and lands on that same foot.

Variations

Hopping in place
Hopping forward
Hopping backward
Hopping diagonally
Hop-kick: Bend your lifted leg in and then kick to the front or side.

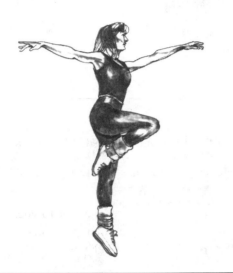

Hopping

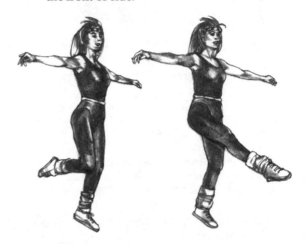

Hop-kick

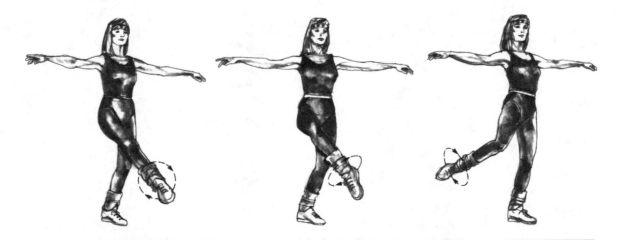

Can-can

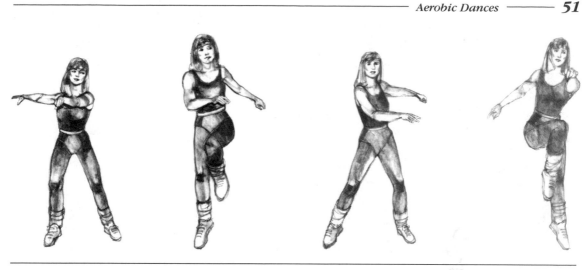

Flea hop

Can-can: Circle your lifted leg from your knee in front of your body. Then bend your lifted leg sideways and circle from your knee. Finally, lift your bent leg behind your body and circle from your knee.

Flea-hops: Take step-hops from side to side.

Leaping

A leap is an aerial movement in which a person moves from one foot to the other. Between the takeoff and landing, the body is suspended in air.

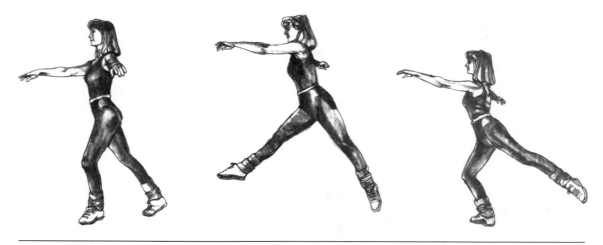

Leaping

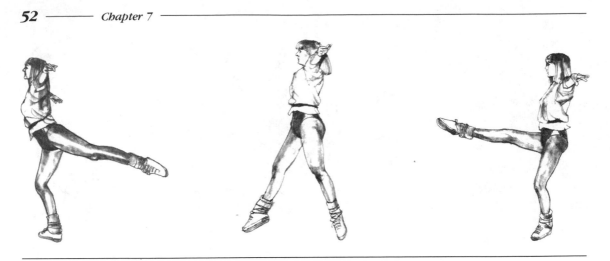

Leaping backward

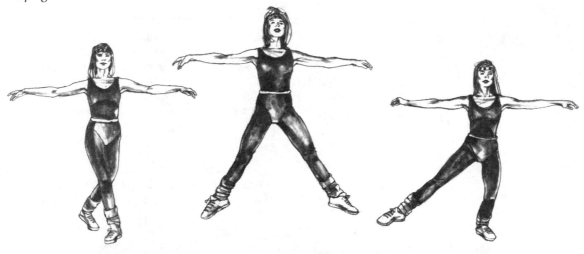

Leaping sideward

Variations

Leaping forward
Leaping backward
Leaping sideward
Leaping diagonally
Rocking: Leap forward onto one leg and then immediately leap backward onto your opposite leg. You can also do rocking from side to side.

Skipping

A skip is a combination of a step and a hop on the same foot, with an uneven rhythmic pattern.

Variations

Skipping forward
Skipping backward
Skipping sideward
Skipping in a circle
Turning

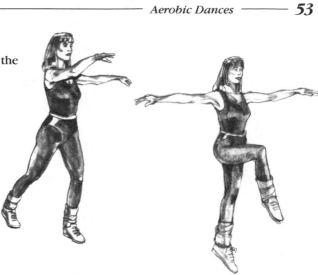

Skipping

Sliding

A slide is a smooth, gliding, step-together step. When performed to its fullest, it brings the body into the air; with the legs together and fully extended.

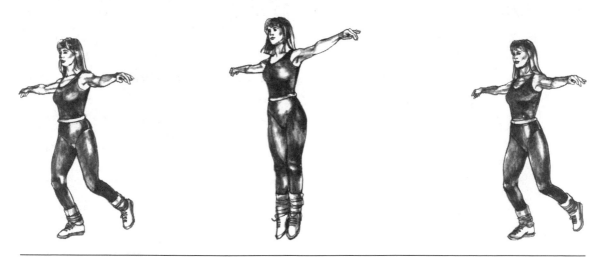

Sliding

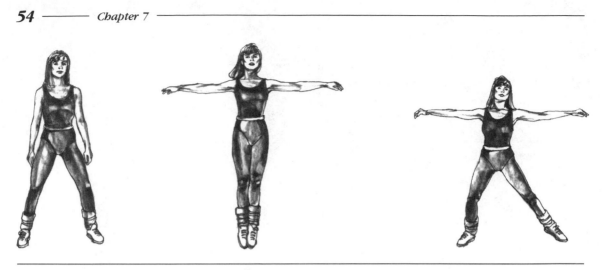

Sliding sideward

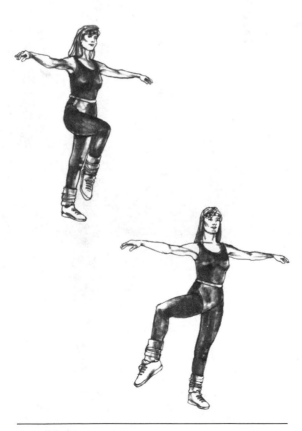

Knee lifts

Variations

Sliding forward
Sliding backward
Sliding sideward

DANCE STEPS

The following movements originate from various dance forms. This brief selection is not inclusive; it is representative of the endless number of dance steps available for aerobic routines.

Jazz and Modern Dance

KNEE LIFTS

Perform to the front or to the side.

KICKS

Perform to the front, back, or side.

KICK-BALL CHANGE

Kick one leg to the front; then step to the rear of your supporting leg, placing your weight on the ball of your foot, with your heel lifted. Your other foot then steps in place, with your weight transferring onto this foot.

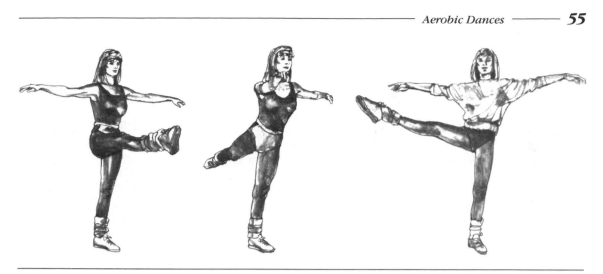

Kicks

PIVOT

Perform the pivot on two feet, quickly changing the direction of your body to face the opposite direction. Both your feet remain on the floor in their positions as you pivot your body.

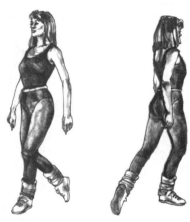

Pivot

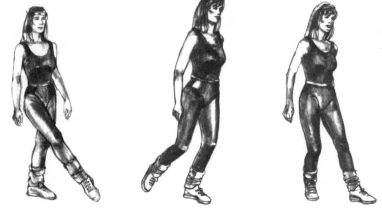

Kick-ball change

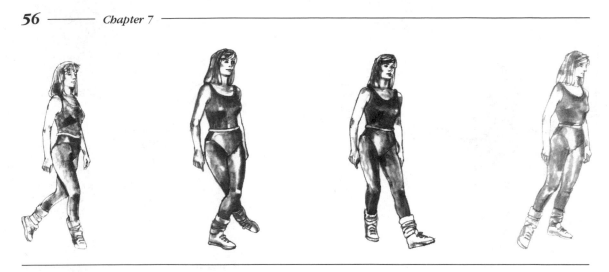

Jazz square

JAZZ SQUARE

The jazz square consists of four walking steps performed in a square pattern.

Folk Dance

SCHOTTISCHE

A schottische is a forward step-together step-hop. Brush your back foot forward, slightly off the floor, on the hop. Make your hop on the same foot as the one you used for the step.

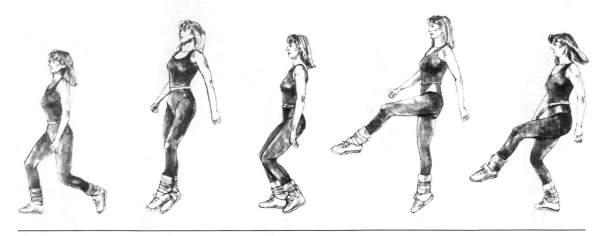

Schottische

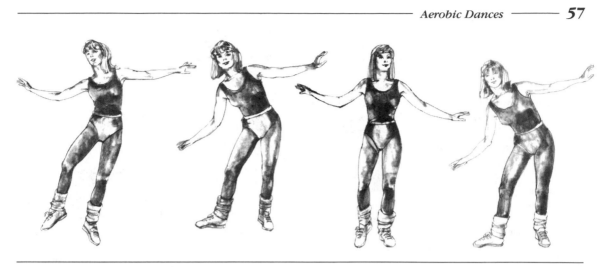

Polka

POLKA

A polka is a hop on one foot with a quick, bouncy step-together step on the opposite foot. The polka can be done from side to side and while turning.

HEEL-TOE POLKA

Hop on your left foot, and place your right heel on the floor in front of your body. Hop again on your left foot and cross your left foot over your right foot, placing your right toe on the floor. Continue with the polka step described above, starting with a left and right step-together step.

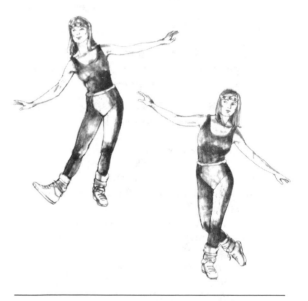

Heel-toe polka

Square Dance

Do-si-doe
Swing your partner

Social Dance

Cha-Cha
Charleston
Monkey
Pony
Waltz

COMBINATIONS OF MOVEMENTS

Just as the locomotor and dance step movements are endless, so too are the combinations of these movements. Listed are a few simple combinations derived from the steps already described. All the combinations can be performed at an intensity appropriate to your fitness level. Kicks can be performed high or low. Running can be geared to a walking pace, and knee lifts can be done without jumping.

3 walks or runs and a hop accented with a snap.

3 walks or runs and a jump accented with a clap.

3 walks or runs with a kick, with arms reaching either vertically or horizontally.

3 walks or runs and a pivot.

Jump reach—jump followed by a hop with your leg extending to the side and your arms reaching diagonally away from your extended leg.

Hopscotch—a combination of a jump and a hop, with your lifted leg crossing behind your hopping leg. This movement alternates hopping feet.

Jump-kick—your kicking leg can kick to the front, side, or back. You can use a variety of arm patterns or perform claps under or over your leg.

Knee lift then jump-kick-jump.

Hop, touching your heel with your opposite hand, then jump-hop combined with a knee lift-jump.

You can perform variations of the basic movements by applying arm patterns. Arm patterns commonly used in aerobic dance include:

Arm circles—make small or large circles with your arms extended to the side and at shoulder height.

Arm scissors—alternately cross your straight arms in front or in back of your body.

Arm reaches—reach up, to the side, or down, or do a combination of all three movements.

Chest stretch—begin with your arms extended to your sides and bent vertically from your elbows, with your palms facing your head and your hands fisted. Bring your forearms together in front of your body. Open your arms until they are in line with your shoulders.

Karate punches—punch each of your arms diagonally across your body.

PRECAUTION

Avoid stretches that violently fling your arms beyond the line of your shoulders, causing the chest muscles to overstretch.

PRECAUTIONS, OR HOW TO SURVIVE THE AEROBIC DANCE CLASS!

Before we describe aerobic dance routines, you should be aware of how to get the most out of your class and avoid complications. Always monitor your heart rate to make sure you are working at your target heart rate. If you have mastered taking your pulse easily, you should continue to walk while monitoring your heart rate. Begin your aerobic workout section at a low intensity; gradually increase and sustain the intensity as you reach your target heart rate. Make sure you are breathing evenly throughout the dances. *Do not hold your breath!*

You should be able to talk while performing the dances. If you are unable to carry on a conversation, you are working too hard. Make sure you *land with your knees bent* on all jumps, hops, leaps, and other aerial movements. Do *not* land with straight legs. Do not perform jogs and runs flat-footed. Your landing must be cushioned by rolling through your foot. Never come to a complete stop during the aerobic section of class except in the event of injury. Slow down to a walking pace if you are out of breath.

Slow down immediately if you feel a side stitch or leg cramps. If the cramp does not stop after you slow the pace, stop and stretch and/or massage the area in pain. If you injure yourself during the dances, seek first aid attention immediately. *Stop* if you feel chest pain, irregular heart rate rhythm, dizziness, or nausea.

Aerobic dance is a time to strive toward your physical fitness goals; it is also a time to have fun. Overload, but do not overdo. Remember, this is not a competition; success means to *keep moving!*

AEROBIC DANCE ROUTINES

Aerobic dance routines are the main challenge and excitement of the aerobic dance class because they enable the aerobic dancers to "dance their hearts out." Aerobic dance routines are performed to popular songs that have a steady beat and lively tempo. The steps and movements are usually counted and choreographed in beats of 8: for example, jog 8 counts, jump 8 counts, hop and kick 8 counts, and so on.

A *phrase* of aerobic dance movements is a combination of two or more sets of 8 counts; thus you have 16, 24, 32, and so on counts of music. The choreography of an aerobic dance consists of several movement phrases repeated many times throughout the dance. A change in phrase in an aerobic dance routine is often determined by the music. For example, a phrase is performed and repeated every time the chorus of a song is repeated. A different phrase is used for the verse, instrumental, and/or introductory part of the music. This division of music gives continuity to the dance and makes it easy for the dancers to remember and follow.

Most aerobic dance routines are performed with the leader at the front of the class and the group facing the leader, but variations of group formations adds novelty to the daily workout regimes. Dances can be performed in a circle, with a partner, or in two lines facing each other (such as the Virginia Reel). Group interaction can add much energy to the class and encourage a sense of classroom community. The instructor should not always be performing with the class; in addition to leading aerobic dance routines, it is the instructor's responsibility to correct posture and alignment, assist students with the execution of steps, and to monitor, as much as possible, individual pace.

CHOREOGRAPHING AN AEROBIC DANCE ROUTINE

The aerobic dance routine must be vigorous enough to sustain your pulse at its target range. Although this is the most important requirement of an aerobic dance routine, the routine should also be fun to perform, with a variety of easy-to-remember movements and dance steps. After all, during the aerobic dance routine, your main goal is to keep moving!

Choreographing an aerobic dance routine follows certain logical steps: selecting the music, analyzing the music, and developing dance movements suitable to the music.

Music Selection

The selection of music is the first decision. It is vital that the music inspires movement because it is the basic motivation for an aerobic dance. The music should be upbeat with a steady tempo.

Music Analysis

Once you have selected the music, listen to the piece several times. When you are familiar with the music, divide it into musical sections: introduction, verse, chorus, instrumental, and ending. Count the measures (8 beats to a measure) in each section, and keep a record of the number of measures per section. Example:

Section	Measures
Introduction	4
Chorus	4
Verse	6
Chorus	4
Instrumental	8
Chorus	4
Verse	6
Chorus	4
Ending	2

Movement Selection

After analyzing the music, experiment by trying various dance steps to a musical section. Select a sequence of steps that lets the choreography move continuously and that can be altered in intensity so your target heart rate will be sustained. Remember that you can create variation in the dance steps by performing the movements in different spatial patterns and directions, combining them with various arms patterns, or by adding accents with claps and snaps.

With your favorite music and combination of aerobic dance movements and steps, you can easily develop your own aerobic dance routine. Two complete aerobic routines are now outlined. You can alter the choreography of these sample routines by adding or deleting repetitions of the movement phrases as suitable to other musical selections.

Aerobic Dance Routine 1

Steps	Repetitions	Counts
INTRODUCTION		
1. Crossover jumping jacks	12 times	2 each (total: 24 counts)
2. Jump and clap	4 times	1 each (total: 4 counts)
3. 3 runs and a hop and clap anywhere in the room	4 times	4 in combination (total: 16 counts)
VERSE		
1. Jump-kicks: kick front, knee lift, kick side, kick front; right, left, right, left	4 times full pattern	8 in combination (total: 32 counts)
2. Jump lunge sideward with arm punches	4 times, alternate sides	2 each (total: 8 counts)
3. 3 runs and pivot	2 times	4 in combination (total: 8 counts)
4. Repeat jump lunges	4 times, alternate sides	2 each (total: 8 counts)
5. Repeat 3 runs and pivot	2 times	4 in combination (total: 8 counts)
CHORUS		
1. Jump reach	4 times	2 each (total: 8 counts)
2. 3 runs and a jump clap forward, then backward	1 time	8
3. Repeat jump reaches	4 times	2 each (total: 8 counts)
4. Repeat 3 runs and clap	1 time	8
5. 3 turning walks and a clap	2 times, alternate right and left	4 each (total: 8 counts)
6. Jump and a clap	4 times	2 each (total: 8 counts)
7. 3 turning walks and a clap	2 times, alternate right and left	4 each (total: 8 counts)
8. Jump and clap	2 times	2 each (total: 4 counts)

Aerobic Dance Routine 2

Steps	Repetitions	Counts
INTRODUCTION		
1. Flea hop	4 times	8 each (total: 32 counts)
VERSE A		
1. Hopscotch	4 times	2 each (total: 8 counts)
2. 3 runs and pivot	2 times	4 in combination (total: 8 counts)

Steps	Repetitions	Counts
3. Jump-kick and clap under leg; jump-kick and clap over leg	4 times, alternate legs	4 in combination (total: 16 counts)
4. ⎫ 5. ⎬ Repeat verse steps 1, 2, and 3. 6. ⎭		

CHORUS A

Steps	Repetitions	Counts
1. Side leap right	3 times	2 each (total: 6 counts)
and		
Jump clap	2 times	1 each (total: 2 counts)
2. Side leap left	3 times	2 each (total: 6 counts)
and		
Jump clap	2 times	1 each (total: 2 counts)
3. Pony	8 times	2 each (total: 16 counts)
4. Repeat side leaps right	3 times	2 each (total: 6 counts)
and		
Jump clap	2 times	1 each (total: 2 counts)
5. Repeat side leap and	3 times, 8 counts	2 each (total: 6 counts)
jump clap		1 each (total: 2 counts)

VERSE B

Repeat verse A steps 1 through 6

CHORUS B

Repeat chorus A steps 1 through 5

INSTRUMENTAL A

Steps	Repetitions	Counts
1. Flea hop	4 times	8 each (total: 32 counts)
2. Knee lift-jump-kick-jump	8 times full pattern: right, left, right, left, etc.	4 in combination (total: 32 counts)

VERSE C

Repeat verse A steps 1 through 6

CHORUS C

Repeat chorus A steps 1 through 5

INSTRUMENTAL B

Repeat instrumental A steps 1 and 2

END

Steps	Repetitions	Counts
Jog in a big group circle	32 times	1 each (total: 32 counts)

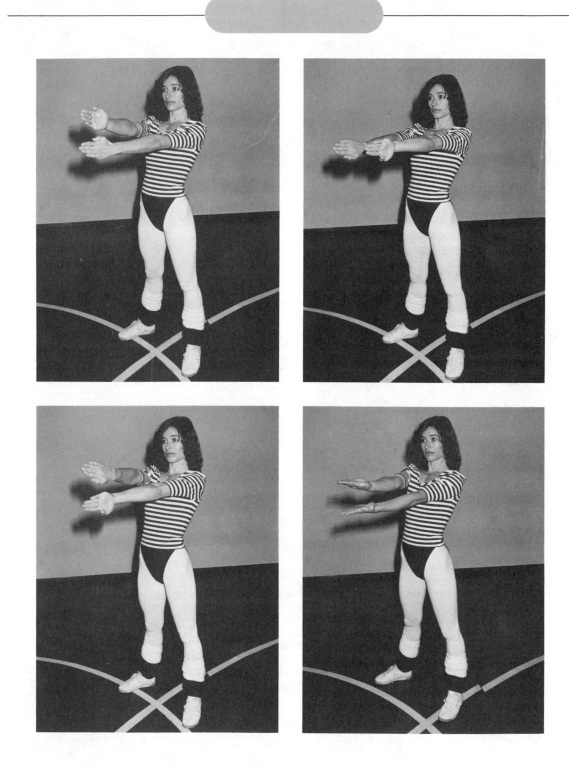

Body
Toning

Chapter

The body toning phase of the aerobic dance program promotes strength and flexibility. During this phase, equal time must be devoted to all the body's muscle groups (Figure 8-1). This session of the class is approximately 15 to 20 minutes long; this time may vary, depending upon an individual instructor's format. Exercises to work specific groups of the body (arms, waist, abdomen, legs, and buttocks) should be blended into the workout with smooth transitions to make the body toning phase more enjoyable. The body toning format emphasizes exercises for one body area at a time.

Muscle tone is a natural tension within a muscle, even when the muscle is relaxed. Muscular contraction, the tightening or shortening of a muscle, will contour and tone muscles. Muscles that are not used regularly will atrophy and look loose and flabby. Exercises that contract and strengthen the muscles give the figure shape and form. Strengthening and toning exercises are those that are performed against a force or resistance; that resistance may be in the form of pushing, pulling, or lifting your own body part or a weight.

To complement the strengthening exercises, flexibility exercises are included in the body toning phase of the workout. These exercises should complement the toning exercises by stretching previously worked muscles. For maximum flexibility, the muscles must be stretched and worked through a full range of motion. Stretching exercises may include any of those described in Chapters 6 and 9. The combination of strengthening and stretching exercises in the body toning phase of the aerobic workout is the ideal format for improving muscle tone and aesthetic appearance. During this phase you can use hand or ankle weights if you wish, to apply overload without increasing repetitions.

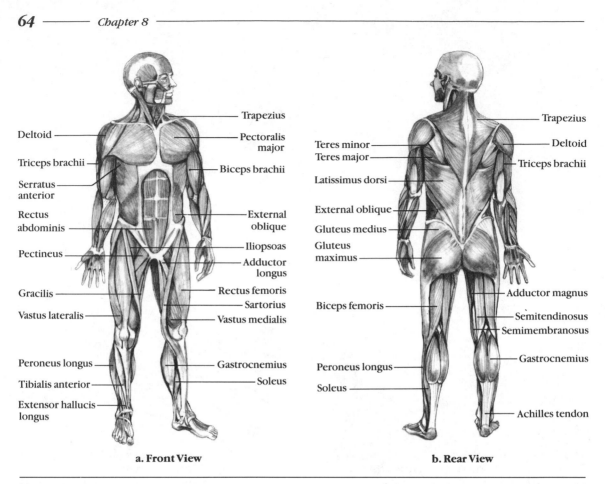

a. Front View

Deltoid
Triceps brachii
Serratus anterior
Rectus abdominis
Pectineus
Gracilis
Vastus lateralis
Peroneus longus
Tibialis anterior
Extensor hallucis longus

Trapezius
Pectoralis major
Biceps brachii
External oblique
Iliopsoas
Adductor longus
Rectus femoris
Sartorius
Vastus medialis
Gastrocnemius
Soleus

b. Rear View

Teres minor
Teres major
Latissimus dorsi
External oblique
Gluteus medius
Gluteus maximus
Biceps femoris
Peroneus longus
Soleus

Trapezius
Deltoid
Triceps brachii
Adductor magnus
Semitendinosus
Semimembranosus
Gastrocnemius
Achilles tendon

Figure 8-1 *Muscular system.*

BODY TONING EXERCISES

Arms

Major Muscle Groups

Triceps brachii
Trapezius
Biceps brachii
Deltoid

SKY REACH

In a standing position with your feet shoulder width apart, reach both your arms upward, with

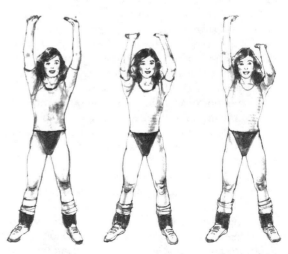

Sky reach

your hands flexed. Bend your elbows, keeping your arms over your head and your hands flexed, and then straighten your arms in a pulsing motion, repeating the "sky reach" several times. You can also perform the sky reach by alternating your arms.

SIDE PUSH

In a standing position with your feet shoulder width apart, extend your arms sideward and to shoulder height, with your hands flexed. Bend your elbow, pulling your flexed hand close to your shoulders. Push your arms back out to the sides. Repeat the pull/push motion several times.

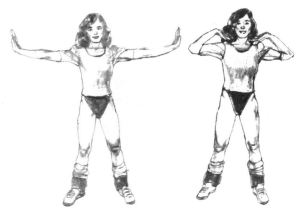

Side push

FORWARD PUSH

In a standing position with your feet shoulder width apart, extend your arms forward from your chest and at shoulder height, with your hands flexed. Bend your elbows, pulling your flexed hands into your chest. Push your hands forward, straightening your arms. Repeat the push/pull motion several times. You can also do the forward push by alternating arms.

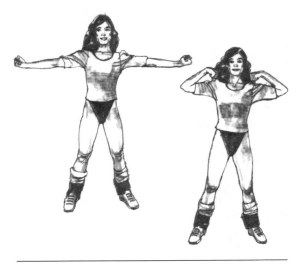

Biceps flexor

BICEPS FLEXOR

In a standing position with your feet shoulder width apart, extend your arms sideward and at shoulder height, with your palms up. Fold your hands into fists. Bend your elbows, pulling your hands close to your shoulders. Extend your arms back to your sides. Repeat the bend/extension motion several times. You can also do the biceps flexor by alternating arms.

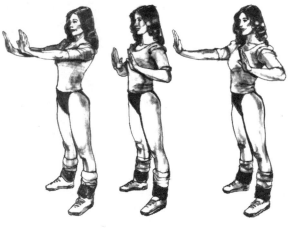

Forward push

FOREARM FOLD

In a standing position with your feet shoulder width apart, extend your arms sideward and at shoulder height, with your palms down. Bend your elbows, folding your forearms toward your chest with your palms turned inward. Extend your arms back out to your sides. Repeat the fold/extension motion several times. You can also perform the forearm fold by alternating arms.

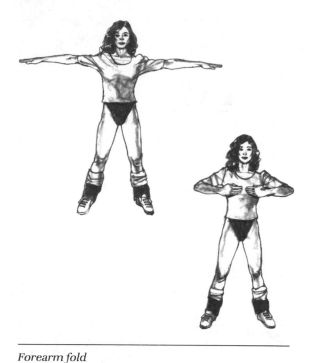

Forearm fold

ARM SCISSORS

In a standing position with your feet shoulder width apart, extend your arms forward from your chest and at shoulder height, with your palms down. "Scissor" your arms by alternately crossing one arm atop the other. To exercise all muscles of the arms, vary the position of your palms: palms up,

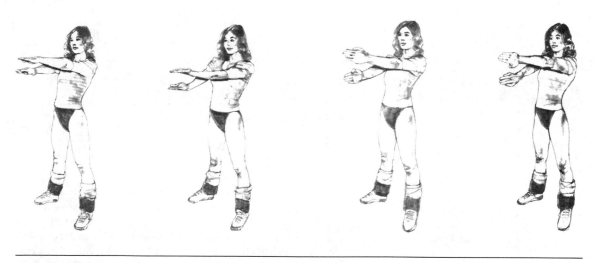

Arm scissors

palms in, palms out. The arm scissors also exercises muscles of the chest (more or less), depending upon the position of your palms.

ARM CIRCLES
FORWARD AND REVERSE

In a standing position with your feet shoulder width apart, extend your arms sideward, with your palms down. Rotate your arms forward in circular motions, progressing from small to larger circles. Reverse the circular direction. You can also perform arm circles with your palms up or out or your hands flexed or held in a fist.

Chest, Ribcage, and Waist

Major Muscle Groups

Pectoralis major; Pectoralis minor (deep muscle)
Serratus anterior
Trapezius
External obliques
Teres, major and minor

Chest

MODIFIED PUSH-UP

Lie prone on the floor. Place your hands under your shoulders, with your fingers facing forward. Keep your feet together, legs bent at your knees. Keep your body in a straight plane from your knees

Arm circles

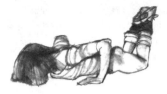

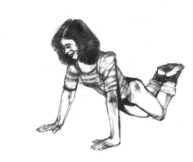

Modified push-up

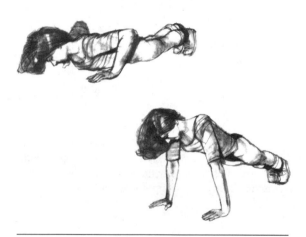

Push-up

to your head as you push your upper body off the floor until both your arms are completely straight. Lower your body back to the floor, maintaining a straight plane. Repeat the modified push-up several times. The modified push-up strengthens the arms as well as the chest muscles.

PUSH-UP

Lie prone on the floor. Place your hands under your shoulders, with your fingers facing forward. Keep your feet together and flexed, with your body weight on the balls of your feet. Keep your body straight, abdominals and hip muscles contracted, as you push up until both your arms are straight. Lower your body halfway to the floor by bending your elbows, keeping your weight equally distributed on your hands and the balls of your feet. Repeat the push-up several times. The push-up strengthens the arms as well as the chest muscles.

———— PRECAUTIONS ————

- · To prevent placing undue strain on the vertebrae of your lower back, do not let your lower back arch.
- · Do not raise your buttocks to dip your chin.

ARM CHEST CROSS

Stand with your feet shoulder width apart, arms extended sideward and at shoulder height, with your palms down. Crisscross your arms in front of your body at waist height. Open your arms out to your sides. Repeat crisscrossing your arms in front of your body, progressively raising your arms until they crisscross above your head. Then continue crisscrossing your arms, lowering them back to waist level.

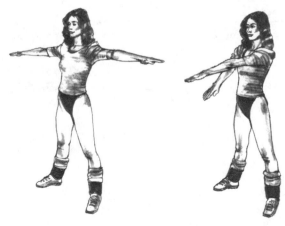

Arm chest cross

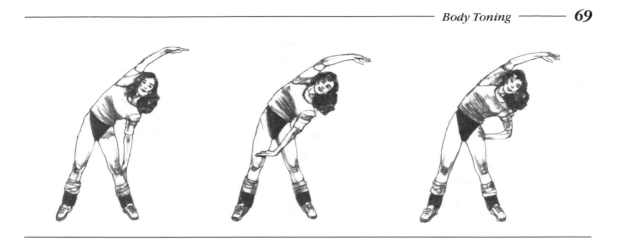

Waist bend

Waist and Ribcage

WAIST BEND

Stand with your feet shoulder width apart and extend your arms sideward and at shoulder height. Bend your upper body to your left, keeping your lower body stationary. Your right arm reaches overhead. Your left arm may reach down your left leg or across your lower body, or you may keep the arm stationary, with your hand on your hip. Repeat the waist bend several times; reverse and perform the waist bend to the right.

SIDE PULLS

Stand with your feet shoulder width apart, with your hands crossed at your wrist in front of your body at waist height. Bend sideways to your right as your right arm reaches down and out to the right while your left elbow bends and lifts up, higher than your left shoulder. Return to the starting position. Repeat side pulls several times on both sides of your body.

Abdominal Muscles

Major Muscle Groups

Obliques, external and internal
Rectus abdominus
Iliopsoas

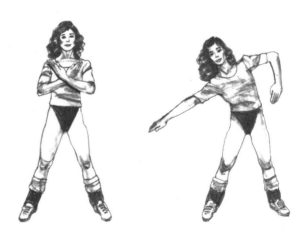

Side pull

HALF SIT-UP

Lie on your back, clasp your hands behind your head, and keep your elbows back. Bend your knees, placing the soles of your feet firmly on the floor. Take a deep breath. Exhale and then contract your abdominals and press your lower back to the floor as you sit up halfway, lifting your head and shoulders off the floor. Release the contraction and lower yourself to the floor.

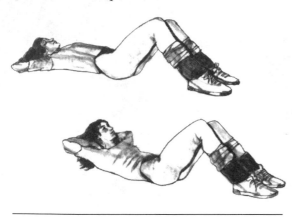

Half sit-up

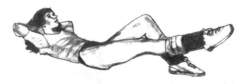

One-leg straight position

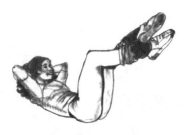

Two-leg half sit-up

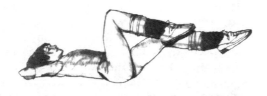

Bicycle

ONE-LEG STRAIGHT POSITION HALF SIT-UP

Lie on your back, clasp your hands behind your head, and keep your elbows back. Lift one leg, straight, off the floor. Proceed with the half sit-up. Now perform the exercise by lifting your other leg off the floor.

TWO LEG HALF SIT-UP

Lie on your back, clasp your hands behind your head, and keep your elbows back. Lift both your legs, with your knees bent, off the floor. Proceed with the half sit-up.

PRECAUTIONS

- To reduce possible use of the lower back muscles, it is important in all half sit-up positions to press down your abdominals, to keep your sacrum on the floor before lifting your shoulders.
- When performing all half sit-ups, avoid placing additional stress or strain on your neck.
- If your abdominal muscles start to quiver and/or you feel yourself lifting and jerking to get up, instead of curling your back, *stop.* Such movements indicate that the abdominal muscles are tired; work will be transferred to lower back muscles, possibly causing lower back pain.

BICYCLE

Lie on your back with your knees bent and lifted off the floor. "Bicycle" your legs.

PRECAUTIONS

- Do not force your neck to flex; doing so may damage the ligaments of your neck.
- Do *not* perform the bicycle in a shoulder stand position, that is, with your neck bearing your body weight.
- Contract your stomach while performing the bicycle.
- Do not let your lower back arch off the floor.

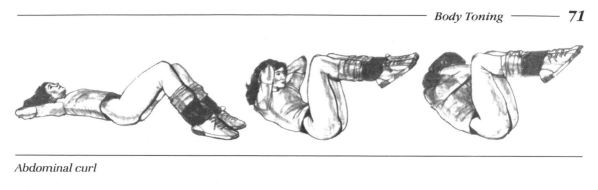

Abdominal curl

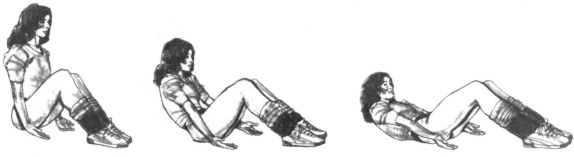

Abdominal curl-down

ABDOMINAL CURLS

Lie on your back, bend your legs, clasp your hands behind your head, and keep your elbows back. Lift your bent legs off the floor and then lift your head and shoulders off the floor until your elbows touch your knees. Release your torso

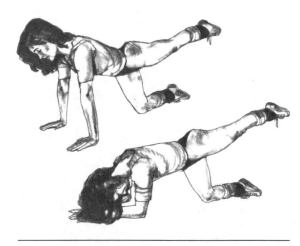

Starting position for leg-lift exercises

slightly away from your knees, but do *not* return to the floor. Repeat the abdominal curl. Exhale with each lift, keeping your abdominal muscles contracted.

ABDOMINAL CURL-DOWN

Begin in a sitting position, with your knees bent and your feet flat on the floor. Relax your arms at the sides of your body. Slowly lower your torso to the floor by rounding your back, contracting your stomach muscles, and placing one vertebrae at a time on the floor. End in a lying position.

Hips and Buttocks

Major Muscle Groups

Gluteus maximus
Gluteus medius
Iliopsoas

Starting position for the leg lift exercises: On your hands and knees, lift one leg so it extends straight behind you, at hip level. Lower your head by bending your elbows and leaning forward, placing your body weight over your forearms.

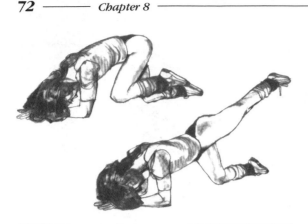

Bent leg lift and extension

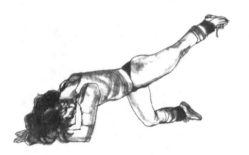

Straight leg lift

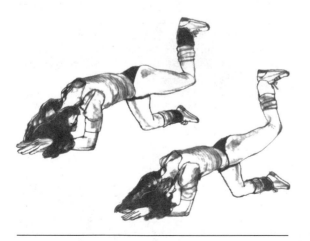

Bent knee leg lift

BENT LEG LIFT AND EXTENSION

From the starting position, bring the knee of your extended leg into your chest, and then extend your leg behind you, returning your leg to hip level. Repeat the exercise with your other leg.

STRAIGHT LEG LIFT

From the starting position, lift your leg up several inches, and then lower it to hip level. Repeat the exercise on your other leg.

BENT KNEE LEG LIFT

From the starting position, bend the knee of your lifted leg with your foot flexed (sole of your foot faces the ceiling). Lift your leg in this position several inches; then lower it to hip level. Repeat on your other leg. This exercise also strengthens the hamstrings.

—————————— PRECAUTIONS ——————————

· Keep your back straight by contracting your abdominal muscles, to avoid placing stress or strain on your lower back.
· Do *not* lift your leg above hip level when you are on your hands and knees. By lowering your head and shifting your body weight to your forearms, you can raise your leg without tilting your pelvis or placing stress upon the lumbar disk.

Back

Major Muscle Groups

Serratus posterior inferior (deep muscle)
Latissimus dorsi
Erector spinal (deep muscle)
Quadratous lumborum (deep muscle)

CAT STRETCH

Begin on your hands and knees. Contract your ribcage and stomach; keep your head down. Hold the position for 10 seconds. Return to the starting position. Repeat the exercise several times.

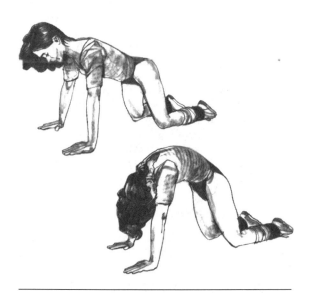

Cat stretch

LOW COBRA

Lying prone on the floor, place your hands on the floor near your shoulders. Straighten your arms while lifting your chest off the floor and arching your upper back. Keep your hips down and lower back relaxed. Slowly bend your arms to lower your chest to the starting position. Do several rhythmic repetitions.

ARM AND LEG LIFT

Lie prone on the floor; lift your arms and legs off the floor simultaneously. Your stomach *must* be elevated off the floor; do so by flattening your lower back with a pelvic tilt (see Chapter 9) and an "abdominal scoop," (that is, pulling in your abdomen). Keep your face parallel to the floor, to avoid hyperextending your cervical (neck) vertebrae.

——— P R E C A U T I O N ———

Avoid the "swan" version (overarched lower back position) of this exercise, which places excessive hypertension in the lumbar area.

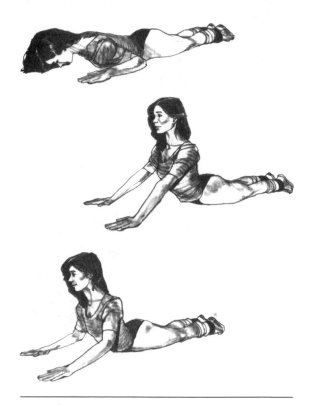

Low cobra

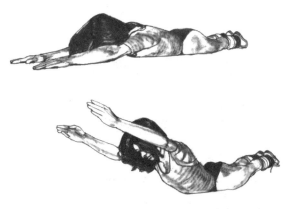

Arm and leg lift

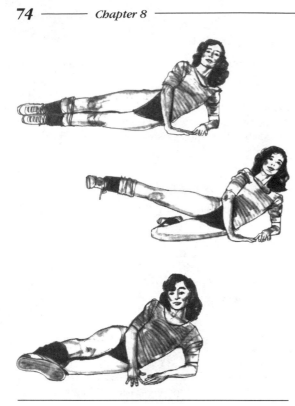

Crossover

CROSSOVERS

Lie on your left side with your head and torso raised, your body supported on your left elbow. Bend your left knee so that your thigh is in line with your torso. Raise your right leg up with your foot flexed; then lower your leg at a comfortable angle in front of you to 3 inches above the floor. Continue to lift and lower your leg in this position with your leg slightly forward. Keep your hips square (not rolling forward or backward) throughout the exercise. Reverse the crossover to your opposite side.

SIDE THIGH LIFT

Lie on your left side with your head and torso raised, your body supported on your left elbow. Bend your left knee so that your knee and thigh remain in line with your torso. Keeping your right leg straight with your foot flexed, toes and knee pointed forward, lift your leg 1 to 2 feet off the floor. (By keeping your knee and foot forward, you cannot lift your leg very high. Avoid turning your knee and foot up toward the ceiling.) Continue to lift and lower your leg in this position. Reverse the side thigh lift to your opposite side.

Thighs

Major Muscle Groups

Hamstrings
    Biceps femoris
    Semimembranosus
    Semitendinosus
Quadricep femoris
    Rectus femorus
    Vastus lateralis
    Vastus medialis
    Vastus intermedius (deep muscle)
Satorius

Medial Thigh Muscles

Adductors: breves (deep muscle), longus, magnus
Gracilis
Pectineus

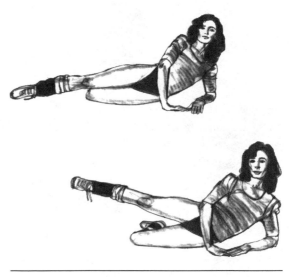

Side thigh lift

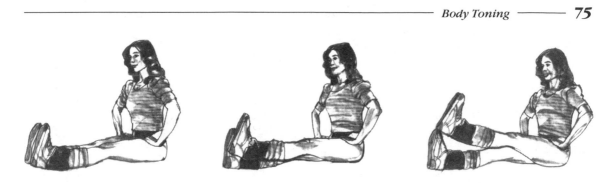

Front thigh lift

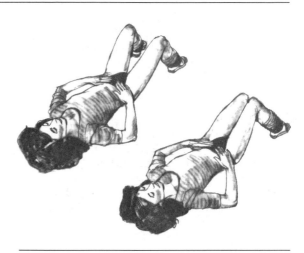

Inner thigh butterfly

FRONT THIGH LIFT

Start in a sitting position, with your legs straight forward and your feet flexed. Lift one leg slightly off the floor (2 to 3 inches). From this position, lift your leg up and down in a pulsing motion several times. Reverse the front thigh lift to your opposite leg.

INNER THIGH BUTTERFLY

Lie on your back with your knees bent, feet apart, soles of your feet firmly on the floor. Close your knees, pressing your inner thighs together. Separate your knees approximately 12 inches. Do not let the soles of your feet lift off the floor. Repeat the close/open motion several times.

INNER THIGH LIFT

Lie on your left side, your body supported on your left elbow. Cross your right leg over your left leg, and place your foot on the floor and your right hand on your right ankle. Keeping your left leg straight with your foot flexed, toes and knee pointed forward, lift your left leg as high as possible. Repeat the exercise several times. Reverse the inner thigh lift to your opposite side.

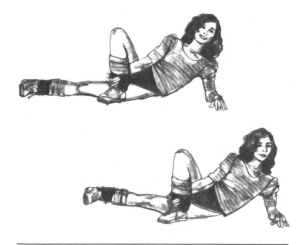

Inner thigh lift

Lower Leg and Ankle

Major Muscle Groups

Gastrocnemius
Peroneus, brevis (deep muscle) and longus
Tibialis, anterior and posterior (deep muscle)
Soleus

Flexors and Extensors of the Toes

Extensor digitorum longus (deep muscle)
Flexor digitorum longus (deep muscle)
Extensor hallucis longus
Flexor hallucis longus (deep muscle)
Flexor digitorum brevis (deep muscle)
Abductor hallucis (deep muscle)
Adductor hallucis (deep muscle)

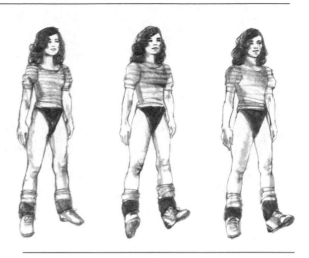

Foot lift

FOOT PRESS

Sit on the floor with your legs straight out in front of you. Have a partner sit in front of your legs and grasp both your feet; your toes should be pointed. Your partner applies downward pressure as you try to flex your ankle. Work through the full range of motion. Do not bend your knees. Repeat the exercise several times (22).

FOOT LIFT

Stand with your back against a wall, with your feet about 12 inches from the wall. Raise and lower your feet several times. You can raise your feet together and/or alternate them (22).

BODY TONING ROUTINES

Body toning routines are made up of many of the exercises in this chapter combined with stretching exercises. Body toning routines should involve all body parts, with smooth transitions from one exercise to the next. A sample routine is described below. (Stretching exercises, which follow the body

Routine for Arms, Ribcage, and Waist

Exercise	Repetitions	Counts per Repetition
Sky reach	32	1 each reach
Forward push	32	1 push
		1 pull
Arm chest cross	4	8 up
		8 down
Elbow clasp overhead (see Chapter 9)	1	Hold for 8
Waist bend–alternating sides	32 right	1 bend
	32 left	1 return to start
Side pulls	32 right	1 pull
	32 left	1 return to start
Arm reach with full torso circle (see Chapter 9)	2 right	4 to circle
	2 left	

Routine for Hips, Thighs, and Abdominals

The following exercises are performed on the floor.

Exercise	Repetitions	Counts per Repetition
Bent leg lift and extension	32 right	1 bend
	32 left	1 extension
Inner thigh lift	16 right	1 lift
	16 left	1 lower
Side thigh lift	32 right	1 lift
	32 left	1 lower
Pretzel (see Chapter 9)	Right-left	16 each side
Pelvic tilt (see Chapter 9)	4	4 lift
		4 release
Abdominal curls	32	1 each
Relax—lie on back, arms above head	1	8

toning exercise section of the routine, are in Chapter 9.) You may vary the repetitions and/or counts of each exercise to fit your individual needs.

IS IT POSSIBLE TO SPOT REDUCE?

Evidence proves that spot reducing is a claim, *not* a fact. The public has been led to believe that blubbery thighs, hips, and arms are merely cosmetic problems. People who promote spot reducing are actually reinforcing a sedentary lifestyle, which is an initial factor in bringing about weight gain and muscular degeneration in the first place.

Exercise of a particular muscle cannot decrease the number of fat cells that lie immediately around that muscle. Also, exercise does not change fat into muscle; fatty tissue and muscular tissue are *not* the same and are not interchangeable. The only way to rid your body of unsightly fat is to reduce the amount of fat or to reduce the size of existing fat tissues.

Working muscles draw their source of energy from fat all over the body. As a result of exercise, fat from all over the body is released, converted into energy, and then used by the muscles. This breakdown of fat to energy is due to the interaction of the nervous, circulatory, muscular, and endocrine systems and is the only way to rid the body of its fatty deposits.

Spot-reducing exercises *seem* to work for two reasons. First, we tend to lose fat first from the area of greatest concentration. Second, when normally unexercised, weakened muscles are exercised, the muscle beneath the fat tissue is strengthened and toned. For example, a woman plagued with what appears to be fat deposits on the back of her arm may really have a weakened triceps muscle. Push-ups and arm-strengthening exercises can help strengthen and tone that muscle, firming the arm area. The circumference of that area may have been reduced as a result of improved muscle tone. As a consequence, it appears that the spot-reducing exercise worked.

But do not be fooled; fat cannot be rolled, shimmied, or shaken off. Saunas and rubberized sweat suits won't rid you of pounds of fat—only water! Only a comprehensive fitness program can help you evaluate your fitness and fat level and help you achieve better overall health and fitness.

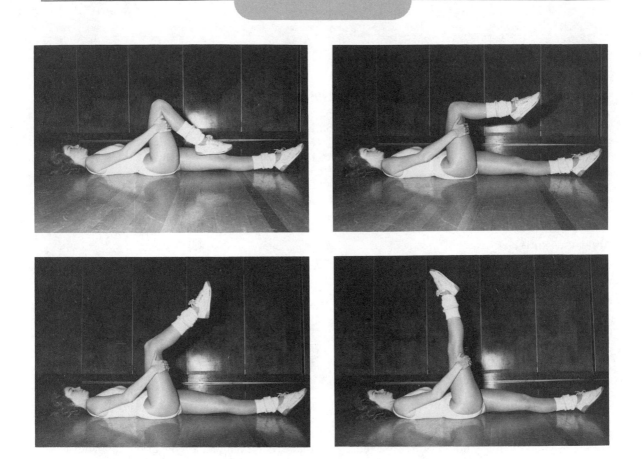

Cool-down

Chapter

9

The cool-down prepares the body for rest, just as the warm-up prepares the body for action. The cool-down is a continuation of the exercises and movements, but performed at a lower intensity, which allows the body to gradually return to its preactivity state. During the aerobic and body toning exercise phases of the workout, the heart pumps a large amount of blood to the working muscles, to supply them with the oxygen needed to keep moving. As long as exercise continues, the muscles squeeze the veins, forcing the blood back to the heart. If exercise stops abruptly, the blood is left in the area of the working muscle. In the case of the aerobic dancer, blood may pool in the lower extremities. Because the heart has less blood to pump, blood pressure may drop, which may cause lightheadedness or dizziness. But a gradual tapering off of activity lets muscles help send the extra blood in the extremities back to the heart and brain.

For the body to have time to recover from the stress of the aerobic workout, at the end of the cool-down phase the heart rate should return to below 120 beats per minute, and sweating should be reduced. The cool-down phase of an aerobic dance class should be at least 5 minutes long. However, the amount of time needed for cool-down varies with each individual. The transition from the aerobic workout to the cool-down phase of the aerobic dance class is accomplished by gradually diminishing the intensity of the exercise and/or slowing down locomotor movements to a walking pace.

The cool-down can also consist of stretching exercises that place special emphasis on the muscles used during the aerobic dances. The following section describes specific stretching exercises and

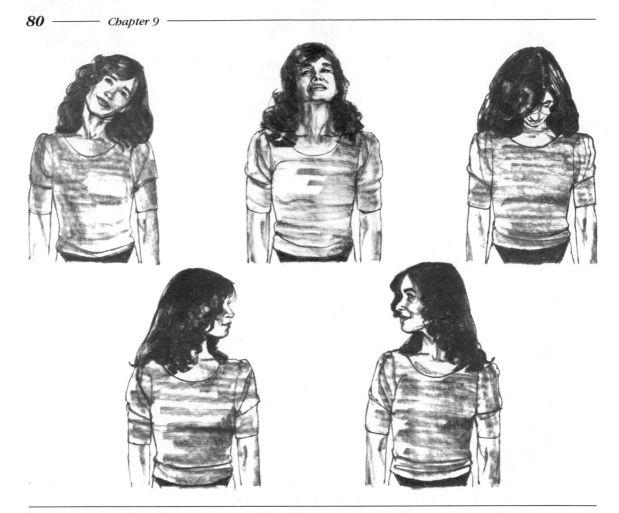

Isolations

their proper techniques. The exercises described in Chapter 6, "Warm-up," can also be used during the cool-down phase of class.

STRETCHING EXERCISES

Neck

ISOLATIONS

You can perform these exercises while standing or sitting: side to side tilt, up and down, look left and right, head circle.

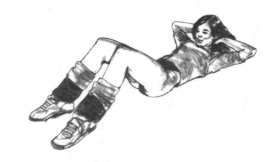

Head raise

HEAD RAISES

Lie on your back with your knees bent, the soles of your feet on the floor, and your hands clasped behind your head. Lift your head off the floor, pulling your chin toward your chest. Hold this position for 4 counts, and then lower your head in 4 counts, stretching your neck away from your spine as your head releases to the floor.

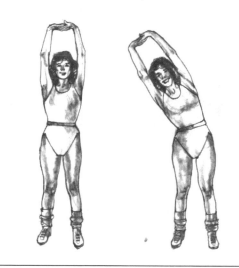

Hand clasp over head

Chest, Ribcage, Waist, and Arms

HAND CLASP OVER HEAD

Clasp your hands above your head and press your palms toward the ceiling, stretching your arms up and back. In this position stretch from side to side. You can perform this exercise while standing, sitting, or kneeling.

ELBOW CLASP OVER HEAD

Cross your arms in front of your body and hold your elbows with your hands. Raise your elbows overhead and pull back. For extra stretch, pull one elbow at a time. You can perform this exercise while standing, sitting, or kneeling.

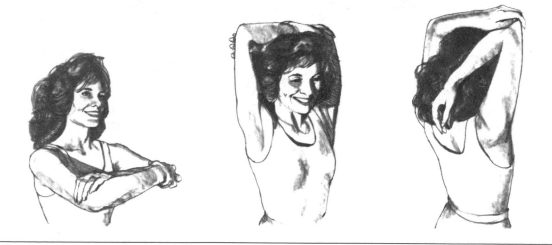

Elbow clasp over head

LUNGE WITH OVERHEAD OPPOSITION PULL

Start by standing in a straddle position with your arms overhead, your left hand grasping your right wrist. Lunge onto your right leg, bending sideward at your waist to the left as your left arm pulls your right arm straight over your head. Reverse the stretch to the opposite side.

LUNGE WITH ACROSS-CHEST OPPOSITION PULL

Start by standing in a straddle position with your arms straight out in front of your chest, your left hand grasping your right wrist. Lunge onto your right leg, and pull your right arm across your chest to the left side of your body. Reverse the stretch to the opposite side.

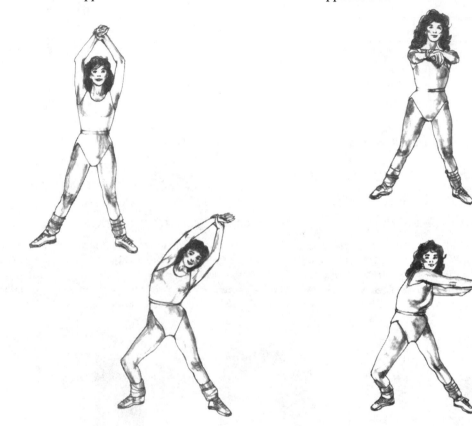

Lunge with overhead opposition pull

Lunge with across-chest opposition pull

Warm-up Exercises That Can Be Used in the Cool-down

Chest stretch
Shoulder circles
Shoulder shrugs
Lateral stretch
Reach stretch
Spinal twist
Triangle stretch

Thighs

DEEP LUNGE

Lunge forward onto your right leg, keeping your left leg straight, both feet parallel. Your body weight should be centered far forward over your lunging leg so that the emphasis of the stretch is on the quadriceps of your right thigh. Extend your arms sideward at shoulder height. Hold the stretch. Repeat the stretch on your left leg.

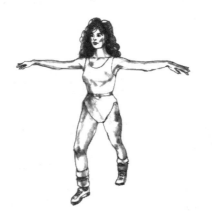

Deep lunge

LYING PRONE THIGH PULL

Lying prone with your legs fully extended, bend one knee so that the heel attempts to touch your buttocks. Grasping the top of your foot, stretch the top of your thigh by gently pulling your foot closer

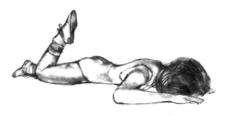

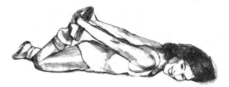

Lying prone thigh pull

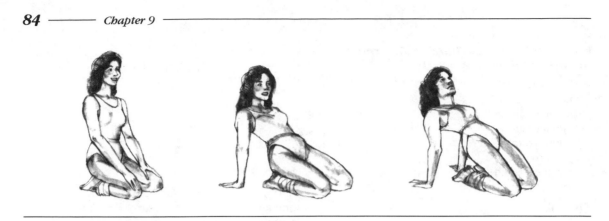

Kneeling thigh hip lift

to your buttocks. Your hipbones should remain in contact with the floor, and keep your abdominal muscles tightened.

KNEELING THIGH HIP LIFT

Kneel with your legs a comfortable distance apart. The heel of each foot should be directly in line with the respective buttocks. Place your hands on the floor a comfortable distance behind your feet. Squeeze your buttocks, and gently lift your thighs, hips, and torso, stretching the tops of your thighs.

PRECAUTIONS

- Do not lift your hips more than 3 to 4 inches off the floor or you might add pressure to your lower back.
- Do not place your hands on the floor in such a position that the chest muscles will be overstretched.
- Do not put your full weight on your knee joint during the exercise.

JAZZ SPLIT THIGH LIFT

Begin in a jazz split: a half-split position on the floor, in which your front leg is straight and your rear leg is bent back, with your heel toward your buttocks. Place the same arm as the straight forward leg in a comfortable position behind your hips. Lift your hips off the floor, keeping your weight on the supporting arm. Stretch the opposite arm over your head for additional stretch of the thigh.

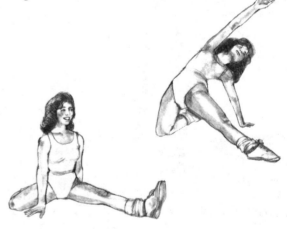

Jazz split thigh lift

Warm-up Exercises That Can Be Used in the Cool-down

Knee lift
Runner lunge

Legs and Groin

LEGS STRAIGHT FORWARD

Sitting on the floor with your legs extended straight out in front of you, relax forward so that your torso is able to move forward onto your thighs.

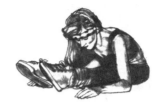

Legs straight forward

PRECAUTION

The legs straight forward exercise is not the sit and reach stretch. The posture of the sit and reach stretch puts much stress on the sciatic nerve by stretching the posterior longitudinal ligament beyond its normal anatomical bounds.

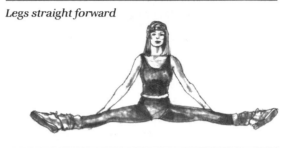

Starting position for straddle stretch

POSITION FOR STRADDLE STRETCHES

Sitting with your back straight, open your legs as wide as possible to a straddle position. Your hips will remain on the floor, and your knees will face the ceiling on all the following straddle stretches.

STRADDLE SIDE STRETCH

Place your right arm from your elbow to your palm on the floor, either inside or outside your right leg. Your left arm reaches overhead while you are stretching your right leg. Reverse the stretch toward your left leg.

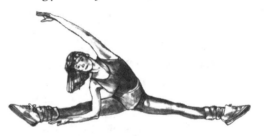

Straddle side stretch

TOWARD THE LEG STRADDLE STRETCH

Twist from your waist as far as possible toward your right leg. Reach toward your right ankle with both your hands, gently pulling your chest toward your right leg. To help keep your back straight, imagine putting your chin on your shin. Repeat the stretch to your left leg.

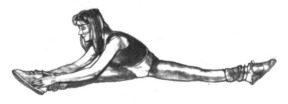

Toward the leg straddle stretch

STRADDLE STRETCH FORWARD

Press your chest toward the floor. Your arm position can vary.

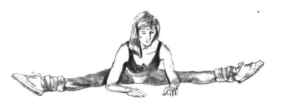

Straddle stretch forward

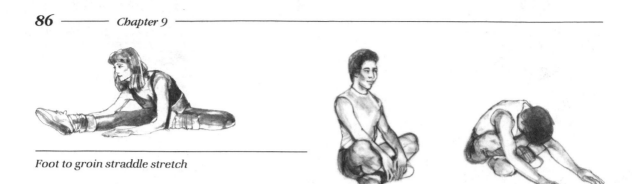

Foot to groin straddle stretch

Indian sit forward stretch

FOOT TO GROIN STRADDLE STRETCH

Bend your left leg so your left foot touches your groin. Relax the trunk of your body over your right leg. Repeat the stretch on your left leg.

PRECAUTION

A groin stretch, commonly called the hurdler's stretch (one leg is bent so that the foot touches the buttocks while the trunk of the body stretches forward over an extended leg), can gradually stretch the ligaments on the inside of the knee (medial collateral ligament) and the tissue of the groin, causing painful fascial groin pulls.

Warm-up Exercises That Can Be Used in the Cool-down

Runner lunges
Parallel forward stretch
Side lunge
Knee lift

Hips

INDIAN SIT FORWARD STRETCH

Sitting with your back straight, cross your legs "Indian" style. Relax your torso forward over your legs, keeping both your hips in contact with the floor. Reverse the cross of your legs to stretch both hips equally.

PRETZEL

Sitting with your back straight, cross your legs Indian style. Lift your right leg and place your right foot on the outside of your left thigh, keeping all five toes in contact with the floor. Keep your back straight, and pull your right knee toward your chest with your left arm while pressing your hip toward the floor. Reverse the stretch to your left leg.

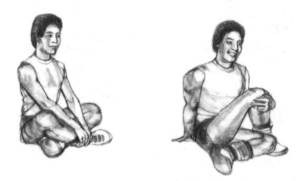

Pretzel

PELVIC TILT

Lie on your back with your knees bent, soles of your feet on the floor, and your hands at your sides. Tightening your buttocks, lift your hips toward the ceiling, approximately 4 inches off floor. Release the stretch, lowering your back and hips to the

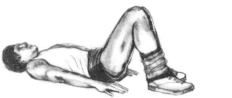

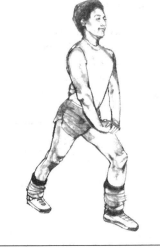

Pelvic tilt

Warm-up Exercises That Can Be Used in the Cool-down

    Hand walk
    Treading

Ankles

ANKLE FLEXION AND EXTENSION

Flex and extend your ankle slowly. You can perform this exercise while standing or sitting.

ANKLE CIRCLES

Slowly circle your foot; be sure to circle in both directions. You can perform this exercise while standing or sitting.

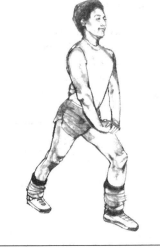

Calf stretch

floor one vertebrae at a time. The pelvic tilt also stretches the thigh and abdominal muscles. *Note:* The pelvic tilt may be done as a body toning exercise by advanced students who understand the body concept of tightening the gluteus and abdominal muscles to support the lower back. As a body toning exercise, the pelvic tilt is done repeatedly in more rapid succession.

Warm-up Exercises That Can Be Used in the Cool-down

    Runner lunges
    Parallel forward stretch
    Side lunge
    Side lunge to the floor
    Knee lift

Lower Leg

CALF STRETCH

In a lunge position, with both your heels on the ground, place your hands on the front lunge leg and continue to keep your back heel on the ground. Repeat the stretch on your opposite leg.

COOL-DOWN ROUTINES

Cool-down routines are made up of many of the stretches described in this chapter. The routines should flow from one stretch to the next, and all body parts should be used. A sample routine is now described; you can vary the counts to fit your individual needs.

Routine for Cooling Down

Stretch	*Repetitions*	*Counts per Repetition*
Pelvic tilt	2 times	8 up 8 hold 8 release
Jazz split thigh lift	2 times right and left	Hold 16 each
Foot to groin straddle stretch	Right and left	Hold 16
Legs straight forward	2 times	Hold 8; release 8
Ankle circles (sitting)	Right and left, 8 times each direction	2 each
Head isolations (sitting)	Right and left, 4 times each direction	4 each
Elbow clasp over head	2 times	Hold 8
Bring body to standing position		8
Lunge with overhead opposition pull	Right and left, 2 times each direction	Hold 4 each
End with deep inhale and exhale	2 times	4 inhale; 4 exhale

PROPER STRETCHING TECHNIQUES

A long, sustained stretch (static) rather than a bouncing (ballistic) stretch is best. Muscles have a stretch reflex: When you bounce, the reflex causes the muscles to react by tightening rather than by stretching.

When you are stretching, go to the point of mild tension. Relax in this position, and hold the stretch for 10 to 30 seconds. Release your position and repeat the stretch. Before stretching a specific muscle, contract the opposing muscle. The reciprocal stretch exercise technique involves an isometric contraction of a muscle group followed by a passive stretch of antagonistic muscles of that muscle group. For example, contract the quad-riceps and then follow with a passive stretch of the hamstrings.

Always perform the exercises with correct body alignment. Two key areas of concern are the lower back and knees. Avoid holding your breath during any phase of an exercise; not breathing indicates a lack of relaxation.

If your body is vibrating or shaking from too much of a stretch, ease up—you cannot relax if you are straining. Not all stretching exercises are appropriate for all people. Anatomical abnormalities and/or improperly performing an exercise can result in injury. If you are performing an exercise correctly but experiencing abnormal pain, discontinue that particular exercise and seek professional advice regarding the problem.

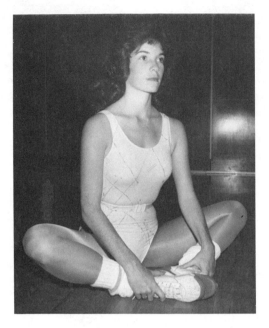
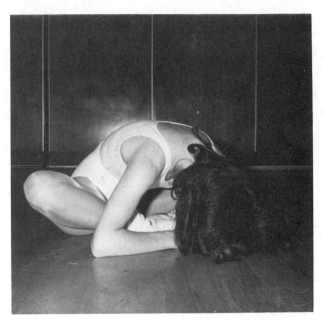

Stress and Relaxation

Chapter

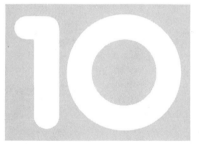

It is impossible to live in today's world without experiencing occasional states of stress. A certain amount of stress is necessary for life to be maintained, for people to resist aggression and adapt to constantly changing external influences. Because stress is inevitable, we must learn to cope with it and to understand when stress has become distress.

Symptoms of abnormal states of stress include restlessness, lack of concentration, tension, anxiety, unreasonable irritability and depression, headaches, insomnia, nightmares, depressed appetite, or increased smoking (7). Everyone occasionally experiences one or more of these states, but it is not normal to be continually beset with them. There are many passive and active techniques to help individuals manage stress. For some of us, relaxation is a skill we must acquire. In our complex world, a life totally devoid of stress is nearly impossible, but by taking the time and making a con-

scious effort, we can achieve the ability to relax. To quote the poet Ovid: "What is without periods of rest will not endure."

PASSIVE RELAXATION TECHNIQUES

Passive relaxation techniques include total relaxation, meditation, and visual imagery. A quiet room with minimal distractions is necessary for following through with these mental relaxation techniques.

Total Relaxation

Lie on your back in a comfortable position. Take a deep breath, counting to 5 when you inhale; count to 10 when you exhale. Focus your concentration on this breathing pattern, mentally dismissing all outside distractions. As you continue, begin to form a mental image of how you look when you are relaxed: Your jaw has dropped; your neck is loose; your eyes are drowsy; your legs, hips, and back are heavy. Your breath is light and easy. Continue this exercise for at least 5 to 10 minutes to experience a state of total relaxation.

Meditation

Sit in a cross-legged position, resting your hands in your lap or on your knees. Close your eyes and totally relax all your muscles. Concentrate on a simple, single word or sound while breathing slowly and rhythmically. If your mind drifts, refocus your thoughts back to the word or sound. Continue thinking of that one word or sound for about 20 minutes. When you finish, sit quietly for several minutes with your eyes opened and then stand up slowly.

Visual Imagery

Lie on your back and get as comfortable as possible. Close your eyes and begin to build a serene world in your mind, such as a mountain lake with the sun shining and a warm breeze blowing. Visualize every detail of the scene, and place yourself in this environment. Continue this visualization for at least 10 minutes. Open your eyes and sit quietly for several minutes and then stand up slowly.

ACTIVE RELAXATION

Find a warm, quiet space with as few distractions as possible. Your body must be in a relaxed position. For the sitting position, rest your hands on your thighs, with your fingers spread, head hung gently forward, and all your muscles relaxed. For the lying position, lie on a bed or the floor. Spread your legs, let your feet roll to the outside, place your arms away from the sides of your body with your palms down and fingers spread. For added support, you can place a pillow or rolled towel under your neck, at the curve in your lower back, and under your knees and elbows (42). Give yourself at least 10 minutes to complete the exer-

cises in a relaxed manner. Your goal is to achieve the sensation of complete muscular relaxation after first experiencing complete muscular tension.

Progressive Relaxation

First lie on your back with your legs straight and your hands at the sides of your body. Relax as best you can.

Next, contract your facial muscles by tightly closing your eyes and clenching your teeth, keeping your mouth tightly closed. Release the tension slowly to the count of 10.

Clench your fist as hard as you can and hold the position for 5 seconds and feel the tension. Feel the tension in your arm? Release the tension very slowly to the count of 10. Repeat this exercise with your other arm.

Flex your feet and tighten the quadricep muscles in each leg. Hold the tension for 5 seconds and feel the tension. Release slowly to the count of 10. Repeat this tension and relaxation process by tightening and releasing your buttock and stomach muscles.

Slow, Controlled Movements for Head and Torso

Slow, controlled movements or large, rhythmical, free-flowing movements also help promote relaxation. Sit on the floor or in a chair in a comfortable position so that you feel no undue muscular tension. Breathe slowly and rhythmically when performing the following movements.

Perform slow, easy neck swings; do not swing your head to the back. Now perform slow, easy shoulder circles. Next, perform slow and easy side bends with your spine, keeping your arms relaxed at your sides. Relax your spine forward and breathe easily.

Exercise can also be a tool for releasing daily tension and increasing your ability to understand stressful conditions. Although experts cannot agree about exactly how exercise works this way, various theories suggest that (1) exercise may simply be a diversion, freeing the mind from stresses that contribute to anxiety; (2) the feeling of accomplishment (of a physical goal) is a factor; (3) exercise reduces muscular tension, thus inducing a state of muscular relaxation. If you exercise to help reduce stress, you must not overexercise, which will re-create a state of stress.

A properly designed aerobic program is a way to reduce levels of stress. However, the program must be within your capacity so that you are not overstressed. Your participation must not lead to staleness or chronic fatigue or cause you to become obsessive about exercise (42).

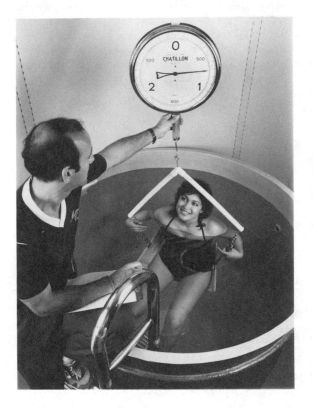
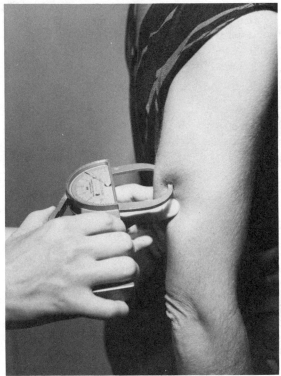

Photograph of hydrostatic tank provided by Alan Rosenberg.

Body Composition

Chapter

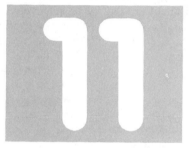

11

How often do we hear the common complaint, "I'm overweight"? Most people are concerned if they are "overweight," but what they should actually be concerned about is being "over-fat." Too many people use scale weight to evaluate their body fitness and health, but we now know that fat can be "hidden" within the body; the scale shows no evidence of fat gain. For example, the average American adult exercises less and eats, drinks, and sits more. As a result, the muscles become less dense, less lean, less "hard." These unused muscles weigh less than they did when they were exercised, and fat begins to accumulate in the body. What used to be "muscle weight" has been exchanged for "fat weight" within the body. This helps explain why we may keep weighing the same but look heavier. Body composition is the body's relative proportions of fat weight and "lean weight."

FAT WEIGHT

There are two forms of body fat: essential fat and nonessential or storage fat. Essential fat is stored in the marrow of bones, in organs like the heart, lungs, liver, spleen, kidneys, intestines, and in the liquid-rich tissues of the spinal column and brain. Storage fat accumulates in adipose tissue, the fatty tissues that protect the various internal organs and that are found in the subcutaneous fat deposited beneath the skin. A certain amount of storage fat is necessary for maintaining health and good nutrition. Women and men need different amounts of essential storage fat: A healthy adult female should have approximately 18 to 22 percent body fat and a healthy adult male 12 to 15 percent. Note that these are not necessarily "ideal" percentages; good athletes often drop below these average figures, and high-performance female athletes often have 10 percent body fat, males 7 percent. Your percentage of body fat should not become so low as to impinge on your stores of essential fat (below 10 percent for women, below 3 percent for men).

LEAN BODY WEIGHT

Lean body weight is the collective weight of the bones, muscles, ligaments and connective tissues, organs, and fluids. During adulthood, changes in lean body weight may occur primarily because the body's muscles are not receiving as much exercise. Although your life may be filled with activity, do not confuse that activity with exercise, which stresses the muscles. You need to regularly exercise your muscles to keep them lean and dense.

Three methods can be used to determine the body's percentages of fat and lean weight: hydrostatic weighing, body composition analyzer, and skinfold measurement.

HYDROSTATIC OR UNDERWATER WEIGHING

The hydrostatic or underwater immersion test is a very accurate method for determining body composition. A person is weighed under water, to determine body density: The more bone and muscle the person has, the more easily the person sinks. Because fat floats, the more fat a person has, the less the person weighs under water.

Underwater weighing is not as simple as it sounds and is usually unavailable to most people because it is expensive and involves sophisticated laboratory equipment. You may inquire about this technique at colleges and universities; many schools use it in their physical fitness education programs.

BODY COMPOSITION ANALYZER

The body composition analyzer sends a mild electric impulse throughout the body and measures body density, determining the percentages of fat and lean body mass. Like underwater weighing, this test can be expensive.

SKINFOLD MEASUREMENT

A calibrated precision instrument called a skinfold caliper is used to measure several predetermined sites on the body to determine the amount of body fat that lies just under the skin. These measurements are computed by a formula to assess the amount of total body fat. Although this method is relatively simple as compared to hydrostatic weighing and the body composition analyzer, it is not as accurate because it gives an estimate of only body fat, not body mass. The accuracy rate is ± 5 to 10 percent of body fat. Because approximately 50 percent of total body fat lies just under the skin and the skinfold test is easy to administer, the method is widely used. It is also a useful comparative test: The original body fat measurements can be compared with new measurements taken at the same sites after months of training or exercising.

Now that you realize that fat can be "hidden" within your body in such a way that you may be carrying excess fat without seeming overweight at all, you can rid yourself of any obsession to look thin. You can also stop using the scale to indicate how fat you are. *Leanness* is what counts, not lightness!

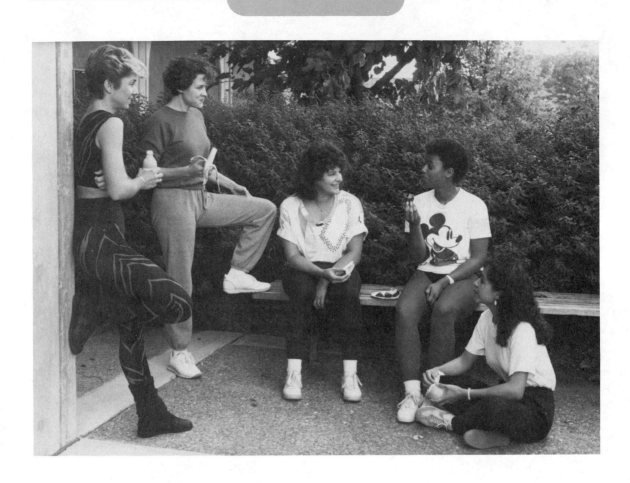

Nutrition and Diet

Chapter

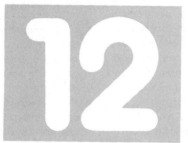

12

Rather than thinking in terms of "diet," which provokes a negative response from most people, you should develop good nutritional habits that you can sustain throughout the rest of your life. The old rule of eating a balanced selection of foods from the basic four food groups still applies.

A nutritionally adequate diet consists of:

1. Milk and milk products
2. Meats, fish, poultry, eggs, and substitutes of nuts and tofu and other soybean products
3. Fruits and vegetables
4. Breads and cereals

To fully understand the basics of proper nutrition, you should also become familiar with the types of nutrients that the body requires and the nutrients' functions.

PROTEIN

The main function of protein is to build and repair body tissue; protein is the basic structural substance of each cell in the body. Protein is found in both animal and plant food sources. The animal food sources are meat, fish, poultry, eggs, milk, and milk products. The protein in animal food sources is called *complete* because it contains the eight amino acids essential to a well-balanced diet. These essential amino acids cannot be manufactured in the body and therefore must be supplied via diet. The plant food sources are lentils, legumes, nuts, cereals, and tofu and other soybean products. This *incomplete* protein lacks one or more of the essential amino acids. Most individual plant foods cannot supply the necessary total protein source; however, when properly combined, they can provide the essential amino acids, such as a combination of rice (grain) with beans (40).

Protein intake should comprise approximately 12 percent of daily total calories. This means 1 to 2 ounces of protein per day, or 0.9 grams of protein per kilogram of body weight (multiply your body weight in pounds by 0.424 to obtain your weight in kilograms) (37). Pregnant and nursing mothers are exceptions to this protein requirement; they should increase their protein intake by 10 and 20 grams, respectively (32).

When the intake of protein is excessive, the process of *deamination*—the breakdown of amino acids to fat—can be very stressful to the body. During deamination, nitrogen is released from the amino acids and quickly converted to ammonia. Ammonia is very toxic to the body and is therefore converted to urea, which is also toxic to the body, but to a lesser extent. For the body to eliminate urea, the urea must be diluted to urine. When the amount of urea is excessive, the body needs enormous amounts of water to dilute it to urine, so much that even consumption of endless glasses of water is not enough. To dilute the urea, the body gets the necessary water from its tissues. The end result is a stressful burden on the kidneys as they overwork to rid the body of urine (38).

Many Americans eat an excess of protein, primarily animal protein. Although animal protein in the diet is a good way of ensuring a balanced supply of essential amino acids, this protein is high in saturated fat and cholesterol and not as easily digested as other forms of protein. Most nutritionists recommend reducing the consumption of animal protein and increasing the intake of plant (vegetable) protein.

FATS

Fats have the highest energy content of all nutrients. Fat's main function is to supply fuel and energy to the body, both at rest and during exercise. Fat has other functions as well: It cushions the body's vital organs, protects the body from extreme temperatures of cold, and helps in the utilization of the fat-soluble vitamins A, D, E, and K (40). Sources of fats include dairy products, meats, margarine, mayonnaise, nuts, seeds, and oils. However, two-thirds of fat intake should consist of nonsaturated and polyunsaturated fats, which are found in vegetables and such vegetable oils as corn, cottonseed, safflower, sesame seed, soybean, and sunflower seed.

Although there is no specific requirement for fat in the diet, there is a need for an essential fatty acid and the vitamins that are the components of fat. Currently, about 40 percent of Americans' daily caloric intake is composed of fat. A recommended dietary goal is less than 30 percent, with the amount of saturated fat in the diet less than 10 percent (42).

CARBOHYDRATES

Carbohydrates supply the body with its primary source of energy, glucose. Glucose (blood sugar) is the product of the digestion of carbohydrates and is stored in the muscles. Carbohydrates also provide fuel for the central nervous system and are a metabolic primer for fat metabolism (32).

Although all carbohydrates have a certain chemistry in common, there is a great deal of difference between one carbohydrate and another. The two general types of carbohydrates are simple and complex. *Simple* carbohydrates—sugars—are maltose, which is found in malt, lactose, found in milk, and sucrose, which is table sugar. When these sugars are ingested, they are converted to blood glucose almost immediately. Therefore, the consumption of simple carbohydrates causes blood glucose levels to fluctuate too quickly, making energy levels vacillate. Table sugar and the refined and processed sugars found in sodas, candy, cookies, cakes, and a realm of other sweetened treats offer no nutrients, are high in calories, and are associated with tooth decay, obesity, malnutrition, diabetes, and hypoglycemia (low blood sugar).

Complex carbohydrates—starches—are the natural sugars found in fruits, vegetables, and grains. Complex carbohydrates are probably the best foods we can eat because they are high in vitamins, minerals, and fiber, which is important for a healthy digestive tract. Complex carbohydrates are also the best source of energy because they convert into blood glucose very slowly and therefore sustain energy output.

Daily caloric intake should include about 60 percent carbohydrates, with about half of that intake being complex carbohydrates (37). You should make every effort to decrease your intake of simple "sugary" carbohydrates, which have no nutritional value, and increase your amount of complex carbohydrates, which offer vitamins, minerals, and fiber.

VITAMINS AND MINERALS

Vitamins help utilize and absorb other nutrients and are necessary for the body's normal metabolic functioning. Vitamins are classified as fat-soluble or water-soluble. The fat-soluble vitamins (A, D, E, and K) tend to remain stored in the body and are usually not excreted in the urine. An excess accumulation of these vitamins may be toxic to the body (32). Water-soluble vitamins (C and B complex) are excreted in the urine and are not stored in the body in appreciable amounts. Minerals are the building materials for tissue and serve as body regulators. Vitamins and minerals are found in all food groups, especially in unrefined, natural foods. A balanced diet provides an adequate supply of vitamins and minerals.

CALORIES

To maintain life and perform work, the body must have energy; the source of this energy is food. The energy food releases is measured in *calories,* or more specifically, *kilocalories.* The number of calories the body needs varies widely among individuals.

Virtually all the calories of energy the body uses are supplied by carbohydrates, fats, and proteins. Carbohydrate is the body's primary energy source. Fats, second to carbohydrates as a fuel source, are utilized if the carbohydrate supply is too low to meet the body's basic energy needs. Protein is an alternate energy source; the body uses protein only when there are not enough calories available in the form of carbohydrates and fats. Protein is rarely used as an energy source; its most important function is to aid the body's growth and repair.

The amount of calories the body requires depends on the amount of calories (energy) it expends. You gain weight if you consume more calories in food than you use during activity. You lose weight if your caloric intake is less than the number of calories your body uses during activity. How much energy (the number of calories) you need in a day depends upon your age, size, and activity level.

As you become involved in aerobic dance, you should intelligently evaluate your body's calorie needs and balance those needs with correct nutritional requirements. To evaluate your diet, keep an accurate record of foods eaten and the number of calories in each food. Your record should show the total amount of calories consumed, with separate categories indicating how many calories were proteins, carbohydrates, and fats. As mentioned earlier, in a balanced diet, 10 to 15 percent of the calories should be protein, 50 to 60 percent carbohydrate, and 30 percent fat. If your record shows an imbalance among categories, make a change in your eating habits (22).

In addition to maintaining a balanced diet, you must have a balance between your total food intake and your exercise output. If your total food intake and exercise output are consistently balanced, you will maintain your weight. If you want to gain or lose weight, either increase or decrease your total food intake while maintaining your output of exercise. In other words, to lose weight you must consume fewer calories; to gain weight you must consume more calories. The best way to lose weight is to combine changed eating habits with a good aerobic exercise program.

A pound of stored fat equals 3500 calories. Thus, to lose 1 pound per week, you must decrease your daily caloric intake by 500 calories; to lose 2 pounds per week, you must decrease your daily intake by 1000 calories:

1-lb fat loss per week = 3500 calories eliminated from diet
= 3500 calories ÷ 7 days
= 500 calories/day eliminated from diet

2-lb fat loss per week = 7000 calories eliminated from diet
= 7000 calories ÷ 7 days
= 1000 calories/day eliminated from diet

Weight loss should involve a weight-reduction program that is consistent and evenly paced. Avoid fad diets, many of which can produce hazardous health problems.

Never eliminate calories totally from one food group, as is called for in many crash or fad diets. If you lose weight quickly, your body does not have enough time to adapt to the lower calorie intake. So you usually gain back the lost weight. And diets that promote quick weight loss by the elimination of water cause dehydration and the loss of important minerals (24). With starvation diets, much of the weight loss includes lean body tissue as well as fat. As a result, the body loses strength and becomes easily fatigued. A nutritionally balanced diet will best help the body respond to the physical demands placed upon it during aerobic dance class. The following sample menus are based upon sound nutritional concepts.

Menu 1

Meal	Calories	Meal	Calories
BREAKFAST		1 pat butter	50
		lettuce salad	30
2 slices whole wheat toast	120	1 T blue cheese dressing	90
1 poached egg	80	1 cup steamed broccoli	60
1 oz cream cheese	105	1 cup peach slices w/½ cup lowfat	
6 oz orange juice	90	yogurt	65
coffee or tea w/1 oz lowfat milk	20		75
	415		750
LUNCH		**SNACK**	
hamburger pattie 4 oz	250	3 cups plain popcorn	165
½ cup creamed cottage cheese	120	or	
1 rye roll	60	1 oz cheddar cheese	100
celery sticks	15	w/4 Triscuit crackers	88
1 medium apple	80		188
	525		
DINNER		Total calories for day	1855 or 1878
6 oz chicken, white meat, no skin	290		
1 medium baked potato	90		

Menu 2

Meal	Calories	Meal	Calories
BREAKFAST		**LUNCH**	
½ cup oatmeal	150	turkey sandwich:	
½ cup lowfat milk	65	2 slices whole wheat bread	120
½ grapefruit	60	4 oz turkey	230
1 slice whole wheat toast	60	1 oz mayonnaise	100
1 pat butter	50	lettuce	10
coffee or tea w/1 oz lowfat milk	20	1 banana	100
	405	carrot sticks	20
			580

Meal	Calories	Meal	Calories
DINNER		**SNACK**	
8 oz perch, meat only	260	1 cup plain lowfat yogurt	130
1 T tartar sauce	75	w/1 T wheatgerm,	100
1 cup cooked brown rice	200	½ cup applesauce, unsweetened	50
8 spears steamed asparagus	30		280
1 cup strawberries	60		
w/1 T light cream	50	Total calories for day	1940
	675		

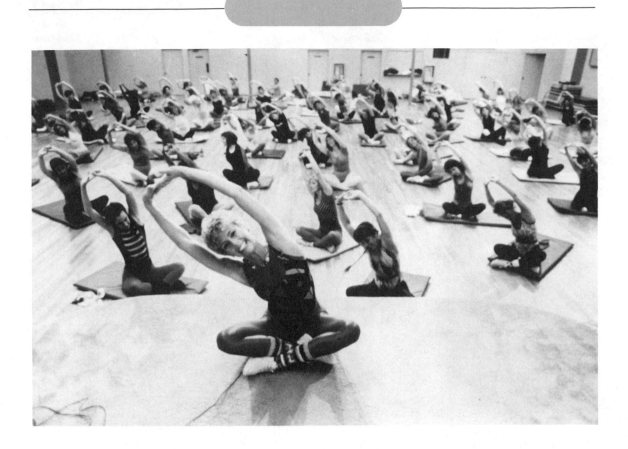

Judi Sheppard Missett, founder of Jazzercise, leading a class.

Take Care of Your Body

Chapter

13

No one cares more about your body than you do, so it is essential that you learn to take the best of care of it. After all, it has to last you a lifetime! Involvement in a sport or recreational activity is not without risk of injury. However, aerobic dance, or any exercise program, is safe if you perform exercises with careful attention to proper technique and take certain precautions. You should recognize and follow the simple guidelines discussed in this chapter.

ASSESS YOURSELF

Evaluate your readiness for beginning an aerobics program. Build slowly and progressively.

FOLLOW YOUR FEELINGS

Do not force yourself to exercise when you are not feeling up to it; on the other hand, do not give in to every little excuse for avoiding your exercise class. A part of all of us would rather sit and relax. Learn to evaluate when to push yourself and when to go easy.

PAIN—A FRIENDLY SIGNAL

Pain is part of our body's language; it tells you when something is wrong. When you have pain, do not ignore it—investigate it. If your discomfort is beyond normal muscle soreness and does not go away or is recurring, seek professional evaluation and diagnosis.

SORENESS

Usually the most common ailment of the aerobic dancer is muscle soreness. When you begin an activity to which your body is not accustomed, you can expect a slight feeling of soreness. There are two different types of soreness. *General* or *acute* soreness occurs during or immediately after an exercise session and disappears in 3 to 4 hours. Acute soreness is thought to be induced by an inadequate blood flow to the exercising muscles (ischemia). This condition causes lactic acid and potassium end products to accumulate; this accumulation eventually stimulates pain receptors. When there is adequate blood flow to the active muscles, these end products are diffused, and soreness diminishes.

The second type of soreness is *delayed muscle soreness,* which increases for 2 to 3 days following exercise and then diminishes until it disappears completely after 7 days. The four popular theories about the etiology of delayed muscle soreness are lactic acid accumulation, muscle spasms, torn muscle tissues, and damaged connective tissues.

The degree of delayed muscle soreness is related to the type of muscular contractions. During eccentric contractions, a muscle contracts as it lengthens. During concentric contractions, a muscle shortens as it contracts. Maximum soreness seems to be related to eccentric contractions (21).

You can help prevent some soreness by:

1. Warming up properly
2. Avoiding bouncing-type (ballistic) stretching
3. Progressing slowly into your aerobic dance program
4. Cooling down properly with adequate stretching

Expect some soreness if you have been inactive before starting your exercise program. Use sensible judgment regarding your body. Do not stop exercising merely because you are a little sore—the soreness will only recur later when you attempt another exercise program.

R–I–C–E: THE RECIPE FOR FIRST AID

Every athlete faces the risk of injury, and the aerobic dancer is no exception. Some athletic injuries merely require self-care treatment. However, other injuries require proper first aid treatment or, depending upon their severity, professional diagnosis and treatment. Apply first aid as soon as you

incur an injury. Immediate treatment quickens the healing process. A simple way to remember the first aid treatment is to keep in mind the initials R–I–C–E:

Rest
Ice
Compression
Elevation

Rest: Stop using the injured area as soon as you experience pain.

Ice: Ice reduces swelling and alleviates pain. Apply ice immediately to the injured area for 15 to 20 minutes several times a day for the first 24 hours after the injury has occurred. Let the injured body part regain its normal body temperature between icings.

Compression: Firmly wrap the injured body part with an elastic or compression bandage between icings. A change in color or sensation in the extremities is from the bandage being wrapped too tightly.

Elevation: Raise the injured part above heart level to decrease the blood supply to the injured area.

You must let an injury heal completely before resuming activity. Once the injury has healed, reinitiate your aerobic dance training *slowly* so there will be no reinjury.

SELF-CARE INJURIES

The following injuries may require first aid treatment. If the injury does not heal with first aid treatment, consult a physician.

Stitch Pain

A pain in the side from running is called a *stitch pain,* which is the result of a spasm in the diaphragm. A stitch pain usually occurs when too much has been demanded from the diaphragm without proper preparation, that is, a proper warmup. A stitch pain may also be due to a lack of oxygen and/or a buildup of carbon dioxide from poor rhythmical breathing. Although many instructors advise running through a stitch pain, this is *not* recommended because more muscle fibers of the diaphragm may become involved and thus increase the strain on the diaphragm.

There are three ways to get rid of a side stitch: bend over in the direction of the stitch, invert the body in the bicycle position, or merely walk. If the spasm releases, gradually increase your speed from a jog to a full run. If the stitch pain persists or returns, *stop!*

Blisters

A blister, caused by friction, is an escape of tissue fluid from beneath the skin's surface. You should not pop or drain a blister unless it interferes with your daily activity to the point where it absolutely has to be drained. If the blister has to be drained, clean the area affected with antiseptic. Then lance the blister with a sterile needle at several points and forcibly drain it. As the blister dries, leave the skin on for protection until the area of the blister forms "new" skin; then clip away the dead skin. You can prevent most blisters by taking sensible care of your feet and wearing properly fitting footwear.

Cramp

A cramp is a painful spasmodic muscle contraction. Muscle cramps commonly occur in the back of the lower leg (calf), the back of the upper leg (hamstring muscle group), and the front of the upper leg (quadriceps muscle group). Cramps are related to fatigue, muscle tightness, or fluid, salt, and potassium imbalance (16). To relieve the pain, gently stretch and/or massage the cramped muscle area. Since muscle cramps can be caused by a fluid and mineral imbalance from profuse sweating, drink water freely and increase your potassium intake naturally with foods such as tomatoes, bananas, and orange juice.

INJURIES NEEDING PROFESSIONAL ATTENTION

More serious injuries that can be incurred from repeated jogging, jumping, and landing in an aerobic dance class are now described. These injuries usually require medical attention.

Shin Splints

Pains over the anterior aspect of the lower leg are generally called *shin splints*. Shin splints usually result from overuse of the muscle-tendon units. The major muscles of the lower leg are contained within fascia (tissue) envelopes. If there is swelling in the muscles, the arterial inflow and venous outflow to the muscles of that compartment can be impaired, causing a slow, activity-related pain in the involved compartment (9).

Several factors contribute to the development of shin splints. One factor is an involuntary collapsing of the arch of the foot, which causes the muscles of the medial longitudinal arch rather than its ligaments to support the bones of the arch. Since the ligaments are intended to be the primary supporters, when the muscles are forced to assume that role, they become overfatigued, irritated, and inflamed.

Another factor is an imbalance of muscular strength on the front (anterior) and the back (posterior) aspect of the shinbone (the tibia) (29). Jogging or jumping on hard surfaces, improper landings from jumps, and improper shoes are also factors contributing to the development of shin splints.

Plantar Fascitis

Plantar fascitis is a direct injury or strain of the plantar fascia, the ligamentous support of the arch of the foot. The injury causes chronic pain and inflames the foot, in particular, the heel. A radiating discomfort may also affect the longitudinal arch. Another cause of plantar fascitis is overuse by putting too much stress upon the feet in relation to the amount of conditioning training and preparation.

Achilles Tendinitis

Inflammation of the Achilles tendon, the tendon of the heel, is common to running sports. Achilles tendinitis is often the result of a single episode of overuse. However, Achilles tendinitis can often be the result of a muscle imbalance of the lower leg.

Muscle Strains

A muscle strain is the overstretching of a muscle, which damages the muscle fibers or surrounding tissue. Often, muscle strains are more complicated than a common *muscle pull*. Once the fibers of a muscle have been damaged, scar tissue forms; scar tissue is not as strong or as resilient as muscle tissue. Most often, injury to the muscles fibers is in the belly of the muscle. However, injury may also occur in the muscle fascia and in the tendons of the muscles that attach the muscles to the bones. Because these areas have limited blood supply as compared to the muscle fibers, muscle strains in these areas take a longer time to heal than do strains in the belly of the muscle (16).

Sprain

More serious than a strain, a sprain is a sudden or violent twisting or wrenching of a joint, causing the ligaments to stretch or tear and often the blood vessels to rupture, with hemorrhage into the surrounding tissues. Symptoms of a sprain are swelling, inflammation, point tenderness, and discoloration. Ankle sprains are the ones most common in aerobic dance. The most frequent is the *inversion sprain,* which results from unstable landings (3). The ligaments on the outside of the ankle joint are the weakest in the ankle and are most susceptible to injury incurred by rolling over on the outside of the ankle.

Chondromalacia Patella (Runner's Knee)

Aerobic dancers may experience a vague pain in the knees when running, leaping, or stair stepping (or walking or running up and down stairs). This pain is characteristic of chondromalacia patella, or runner's knee, an erosion of the cartilage covering the underside of the kneecap or patella. Internal factors that affect chondromalacia are anatomical malalignment of the lower extremities:

Discrepancy in leg length
Abnormality in rotation of hips
Bowlegs
Knock-knees
Flatfeet
Musculature imbalance

The following external factors can also promote the problem:

Training errors, including abrupt changes in intensity, duration, or frequency
Improper footwear
Bad running surfaces (2); avoid dancing on cement floors

Patellar Tendinitis (Jumper's Knee)

Repetitive jumping and landing activities can produce small scars in the patellar tendon, causing pain, tenderness, and inflammation directly below the kneecap. Often, the aching of the knees apparent at the beginning of a workout disappears after warm-up. However, pain recurs when activity ceases. In a worsened condition, pain continues throughout a workout, and pressing on the tendon itself causes pain.

Any sort of injury can take time away from your aerobic training program. Use proper precautions and common sense in initiating your training. If you are injured, remember the simple steps of first aid treatment: rest, ice, compression, elevation; apply the treatment immediately after injury occurs. Seek medical advice for injuries that persist or for any serious injury.

Sources for Fitness Evaluations

Fitness evaluation tests and charts are used at the teacher's discretion.

TESTS

A number of valid tests can be used to evaluate your level of fitness; we recommend the following references.

Endurance Tests

1.5 mile test: Kenneth H. Cooper, *The Aerobics Way,* New York: M. Evans, 1977.

3-minute step test: Y.M.C.A. of the U.S.A.; *3-Minute Step Test,* 101 N. Wacker Drive, Chicago, IL 60606.

Strength Tests

Abdominal strength: Y.M.C.A. of the U.S.A., *Abdominal Strength Test,* 101 N. Wacker Drive, Chicago, IL 60606.

Arm strength: Dorie Krepton and Donald Chu, *Everybody's Aerobic Book,* Edina, MN: Bellwether Press, 1986.

Leg strength: Dorie Krepton and Donald Chu, *Everybody's Aerobic Book,* Edina, MN: Bellwether Press, 1986.

Flexibility

Shoulder lift: Charles A. Bucher and William E. Prentice, *Fitness for College and Life,* St. Louis: Mosby, 1985.

Sit and reach: Charles A. Bucher and William E. Prentice, *Fitness for College and Life,* St. Louis: Mosby, 1985.

Trunk extension: R. V. Hockey, *Physical Fitness,* 5th ed., St. Louis Times Mirror/Mosby, 1985.

Hip flexion and hamstring mobility: Dorie Krepton and Donald Chu, *Everybody's Aerobic Book,* Edina, MN: Bellwether Press, 1986.

Body Composition

Skinfold test: Research Quarterly for Exercise and Sport, vol. 52, 1981.

CHARTS

The following charts are of value to the teacher and student as a means of personal evaluation. Feel free to duplicate these forms.

Student Profile

N A M E _____

A D D R E S S _____

P H O N E _____

Rate your fitness level:

_____ Superior   _____ Fair

_____ Excellent   _____ Poor

_____ Good   _____ Very poor

Previous instruction in aerobic dance _____

Sports/exercise in which you participate _____

Reasons for taking this course _____

Did anyone recommend this course or instructor? _____

Your physical limitations _____

Activity or type of exercise you would like to have covered _____

_____

Your heart rate:

_____ Resting

_____ Target

Do you want to:

_____ Gain lean weight

_____ Lose fat weight

_____ Stay the same

Do you smoke? _____   If so, how many cigarettes per day? _____

List your favorite kind of music, favorite song, favorite singer or group _____

_____

List your interests _____

_____

Body Measurement

N A M E _____

Procedure: Measure each area at its widest part.

Measurements

Area	Initial	After 8 weeks	After 16 weeks
Weight			
Biceps	R L	R L	R L
Chest			
Waist			
Abdomen			
Hips			
Thighs	R L	R L	R L
Calves	R L	R L	R L
Ankles	R L	R L	R L

APPENDIX B
Suggested Reading

AEROBICS AND FITNESS

Allsen, Phillip E., Joyce M. Harrison, and Barbara Vance. *Fitness for Life.* Dubuque, IA: Brown, 1983.

Bailey, Covert. *Fit or Fat.* Boston: Houghton Mifflin, 1978.

Cooper, Kenneth H. *The Aerobics Program for Total Well-Being.* New York: Bantam, 1983.

Cooper, Kenneth H. *Aerobics for Women.* New York: Bantam, 1980.

Getchell, Bud. *Physical Fitness: A Way of Life.* New York: Wiley, 1983.

Greggains, Joanie. *Joanie Greggains' Total Shape Up.* New York: New American Library, 1984.

Miller, D., and E. Allen. *Fitness: A Lifetime Concept.* Minneapolis: Burgess, 1982.

Smith, Kathy. *Ultimate Workout.* New York: Bantam, 1983.

BODY TONING AND STRENGTH BUILDING

Darden, Ellington. *The Nautilus Book.* Chicago: Contemporary Books, 1982.

Darden, Ellington. *The Nautilus Woman.* New York: Simon and Schuster, 1983.

Lance, Kathryn. *Getting Strong.* Indianapolis: Bobbs-Merrill, 1978.

Westcott, W. L. *Strength Fitness.* Boston: Allyn and Bacon, 1982.

FLEXIBILITY

Anderson, Bob. *Stretching.* Blinds, CA: Shelter Publications, 1980.

Benjamin, Ben E. *Sports Without Pain.* New York: Summit Books, 1979.

INJURIES

Arnheim, D. *Modern Principles of Athletic Training,* 7th ed. St. Louis: Times Mirror/Mosby, 1985.

Fahey, Tom. *Athletic Training: Principles and Practice.* Palo Alto, CA: Mayfield, 1986.

Morris, A. *Sports Medicine: Prevention of Athletic Injuries.* Dubuque, IA: Brown, 1984.

Wright, S. *Dancer's Guide to Injuries of the Lower Extremities.* New York: Cornwall Books, 1985.

NUTRITION

Bailey, Covert. *Fit or Fit Target Diet.* Boston: Houghton Mifflin, 1984.

Brody, Jane. *Jane Brody's Nutrition Book.* New York: Bantam, 1981.

Dusky, Lorraine, and J. J. Leedy. *How to Eat like a Thin Person.* New York: Simon and Schuster, 1982.

Whitney, Eleanore Noss, and Eva May Hamilton. *Nutrition: Concepts and Controversies.* St. Paul: West, 1982.

Low-Impact
and Nonimpact
Aerobic Dance

People with hip, knee, and ankle problems often complain about the high-intensity jumping and bouncing that are characteristic of aerobic dance. Low-impact and nonimpact styles of aerobic dance reduce the strain. In low-impact routines, one foot is always on the ground, and the shock of jumps is thus eliminated. Nonimpact aerobics decreases the stress even more because neither foot leaves the ground; all the movements are done by bending and straightening the knees.

Nonimpact styles contain their own injury risk: Bending the knees too deeply can damage the ligaments. The knees should always be directly in line with the toes. Movements should be controlled and smooth, not jerky or bouncy.

In both low- and nonimpact aerobic dance, arm movements are large and continuous throughout the workout. The use of the arms and the large muscles of the legs (quadriceps and hamstrings) causes the heartbeat to rise to an aerobic level.

Any of the steps described in Chapter 7 can be modified to fit into a low- or nonimpact class. Remember not to bounce and to keep at least one or both feet in contact with the floor at all times. Because of the continual use of the bent knee position, the cool-down phase of the class should be sure to emphasize stretching of the quadriceps and hamstrings.

Here are some examples of how to modify aerobic dance steps.

KNEE LIFTS

Bend the supporting leg while lifting the opposite knee to the chest, to the side, or across the body. Straighten the leg as the knee is lowered. The arms can pull down toward the waist from a high position with elbows bending and straightening.

KICKS

Perform the same as knee lifts, but the extended leg will be straight and can go to the front, side, back, or across the body. The arms can push toward the ceiling, to the sides, or in front of the body.

LUNGES

Open one leg to the front, side, or back, making sure it is bent while the other leg is straight. Then bring both legs together, knees straight. The arms can lift and lower as the leg opens and closes.

HOPSCOTCH

With the feet in a wide position, bend both knees; then straighten one leg as you lift it off the ground and bend it behind the supporting leg. The arms can swing high toward the supporting leg or can complete a circle.

JOGGING

Instead of jogging, use a power walk. This is a wide-stride walk done with the knees bent. The arms can punch in various directions.

The main cue you will continually hear in a low- or nonimpact class will be *do not bounce!* But, as in any aerobic dance class, don't forget to *keep moving!*

References

1. Allsen, Philip E. *Conditioning and Physical Fitness.* Dubuque, IA: Brown, 1978.
2. American College of Sports Medicine. "Recommendations and Quality of Exercise for Developing and Maintaining Fitness in Healthy Adults." *Journal of Physical Education and Recreation* 51, no. 5 (May 1980): 17–18.
3. Bailey, Covert. *Fit or Fat?* Boston: Houghton Mifflin, 1977.
4. Benson, Herbert. *The Relaxation Response.* New York: Avon, 1975.
5. Bernard, R. J. *The Heart Needs Warm-up Time.*
6. Bogart, J., et al. *Nutrition and Physical Fitness.* Philadelphia: Saunders, 1979.
7. Bucher, Charles A., and William E. Prentice. *Fitness for College and Life.* St. Louis: Times/Mirror, Mosby, 1985.
8. Cantu, Robert C. *Sports Medicine in Primary Care.* Lexington, MA: Heath, 1982.
9. Cantu, Robert C. *Clinical Sports Medicine.* Lexington, MA: Heath, 1983.
10. Cantu, Robert C., and William Jay Gillespie. *Sports Medicine, Sports Science: Bridging the Gap.* Lexington, MA: Heath, 1982.
11. Clearly, Monica L., Robert J. Moffat, and Kathleen M. Knutzen. "The Effects of Two- and Three-Day per Week Aerobic Dance Programs on Maximal Oxygen Uptake." *Research Quarterly for Exercise and Sport* 55, no. 1 (1984): 172–174.
12. Cooper, Kenneth H. *The Aerobics Way.* New York: Evans, 1977.
13. Corbin, Charles B., and Ruth Lindsey. *Concepts of Fitness.* Dubuque, IA: Brown, 1985.
14. Corbin, Charles B., and Ruth Lindsey. *Concepts of Physical Fitness with Laboratories.* Dubuque, IA: Brown, 1985.
15. DeVries, H. A. *Physiology of Exercise for Physical Education and Athletics,* 3rd ed. Dubuque, IA: Brown, 1980.
16. Dintiman, George B., Stephen E. Stone, Jude C. Pennington, and Robert G. Davis. *Discovering Lifetime Fitness: Concepts of Exercise and Weight Control.* St. Paul, MN: West, 1984.
17. Dowdy, Deborah, Kirk J. Cureton, Harry P. DuVal, and Harvey G. Outz. "Effects of Aerobic Dance on Physical Work Capacity, Cardiovascular Function, and Body Composition of Middle-aged Women. *Research Quarterly for Exercise and Sport* 56, no. 3 (1985): 227–233.
18. Dusek, Dorothy E. *Thin and Fat: Your Personal Lifestyle.* Belmont, CA: Wadsworth, 1978.
19. Falls, Harold B., Ann M. Baylor, and Rod K. Dishman. *Essentials of Fitness.* Philadelphia: SCP, 1980.
20. Fox, S. M., J. P. Naughton, and W. L. Hackcll. "Physical Activity: The Prevention of Coronary Heart Disease." *Annals of Clinical Research* 3

(1971): 404–432.

21. Francis, Kennon T. "Delayed Muscle Soreness: A Review." *Journal of Orthopedic and Sports Physical Therapy* (1983).

22. Francis, Lorna L. *Injury Prevention Manual for Dance Exercises.* San Diego, CA: National Injury Prevention Foundation, 1983.

23. Getchell, Bud. *Physical Fitness: A Way of Life,* 3rd ed. New York: Macmillan, 1983.

24. Goodman Kraines, Minda, and Esther Kan. *Jump into Jazz.* Palo Alto, CA: Mayfield, 1983.

25. Jacobson, Edmund. *You Must Relax.* New York: McGraw-Hill, 1962.

26. Jensen, Clayne R., and Garth A. Fisher. *Scientific Basis of Athletic Conditioning,* 2nd ed. Philadelphia: Lea & Febiger, 1979.

27. Katch, F. I., and W. D. McArdle. *Nutrition, Weight Control, and Exercise.* Boston: Houghton Mifflin, 1977.

28. Kisselle, Judy, and Karen Mazzeo. *Aerobic Dance, Alternate Edition.* Englewood, CO: Morton, 1984.

29. Krepton, Dorie, and Donald Chu, *Everybody's Aerobic Book,* Edina, MN: Bellwether Press, 1986.

30. Lamb, David R. *Physiology of Exercise: Response and Adaptations,* 2nd ed. New York: Macmillan, 1984.

31. Martin, B. J. "Effect of Warm-up on Metabolic Responses to Strenuous Exercise." *Medicine in Science and Sport* 7, no. 2 (1975): 146–149.

32. McArdle, William D., Frank I. Katch, and Victor L. Katch. *Exercise Physiology: Energy, Nutrition, and Human Performance.* Philadelphia: Lea & Febiger, 1981.

33. Moorhouse, Laurence. *Total Fitness.* New York: Simon and Schuster, 1975.

34. Nash, Jay B. "You Must Relax—But How?" *Health Education* 16 (April–May 1985): 9–12.

35. Rasch, P. J., and R. K. Burke. *Kinesiology and Applied Anatomy,* 6th ed. Philadelphia: Lea & Febiger, 1978.

36. Selye, Hans. *The Stress of Life.* New York: McGraw-Hill, 1956.

37. Sharkey, Brian J. *Physiology of Fitness.* Champaign, IL: Human Kinetics, 1979.

38. Simonson, Ernst (Ed.). *Physiology of Work Capacity and Fatigue.* Springfield, IL: Thomas, 1971.

39. University of California, Cardiac Rehabilitation Program. "Things to Know About Your Lower Back." Davis, CA: 1981.

40. Vitale, Frank. *Individualized Fitness Program.* Englewood Cliffs, NJ: Prentice-Hall, 1973.

41. White, J. R. "EKG Changes Using Carotid Artery for HR Monitoring." *Medicine and Science in Sports and Exercise* 9 (1977): 88–94.

42. Williams, Melvin. *Lifetime Physical Fitness.* Dubuque, IA: Brown, 1985.

Index

117